FAMILY-CENTRED CARE

Family-Centred Care

Concept, Theory and Practice

Edited by

**Lynda Smith, Valerie Coleman,
Maureen Bradshaw**

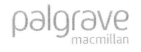

First published 2002 by
PALGRAVE
Houndmills, Basingstoke, Hampshire RG21 6XS and
175 Fifth Avenue, New York, N. Y. 10010
Companies and representatives throughout the world

PALGRAVE is the new global academic imprint of
St. Martin's Press LLC Scholarly and Reference Division and
Palgrave Publishers Ltd (formerly Macmillan Press Ltd).

ISBN 0–333–92293–X

This book is printed on paper suitable for recycling and
made from fully managed and suitable forest sources.

A catalogue record for this book is available
from the British Library.

Printed and bound by Antony Rowe Ltd, Eastbourne

Contents

List of Figures and Tables

Figures

Tables

vii

Foreword

I cannot remember when I last read a nursing text and felt the same sense of relief, at last we have a resource which brings together the mass of concepts, theories and practice issues which are so fundamental to children's nursing. As a teacher and now as an editor, it seemed that everyone writing about any aspect of working with children and families redefined the concepts and arrived at a different place but did little to move us forward. Now the scattered literature is collected together and added to in such a way that we can all learn from it.

The authors of this book provide an historical overview of family-centred care which nicely illustrates how this construct evolved and continues to evolve, along with related constructs such as empowerment, collaboration, negotiation and participation. Locating this evolution in the context of societal, professional and healthcare changes is essential and there are helpful clarifications throughout the book, many of which provide practical models to inform education and practice. What is unique about this book is that it really does take the step of putting theories into practice.

Using case examples and guidelines, the authors clearly set out the behaviours and attributes which facilitate family-centred care, making it appropriate to the family context and to family preferences. Students and experienced nurses will be able to make better sense of the theories as well as learning new ones and looking at old ones from different perspectives. They are helped in these pages to work out where to begin, to develop skills in providing information, building relationships, negotiating care and facilitating parent or family-led services.

In their preface, the editors indicate that the book is designed to introduce the student nurse to family-centred care. One of the failings of our present continuing education provision for nurses is that it focuses on specialist education and fails to develop further the general children's nursing expertise of the registered children's nurse. This book would make an excellent introduction for those wanting to increase their level of expertise in working with children and families at any stage in their careers. We could have carried on for many more years in children's nursing with theoretical debates, refining the meaning of negotiation, empowerment, partnership and the rest. I am very glad that someone identified the need for this book and, having done so, pulled it together in such an accessible and practical way.

ANNE CASEY
RSCN, RGN, MSc, DipNEd
Editor, 'Paediatric Nursing'

Preface

The impetus to write this book came from our extensive experiences both in clinical practice and teaching students. Students often find it difficult to apply the theoretical components of family-centred care into everyday practice. Children's nursing textbooks have tended to focus on the conceptual elements of family-centred care rather than on practical application and skills development. It is our intention to redress this imbalance by providing a comprehensive text that specifically addresses both theoretical and practice components of family-centred care. The text will be valuable to student nurses and qualified nurses working with children and families both in hospital and community settings.

Family-Centred Care: Concept, Theory and Practice is a contemporary text that acknowledges the challenges, including legal ones, faced by nurses in facilitating the concept and provides support for the development of skills required for its implementation. This text values the importance of the practical skills of empowerment, negotiation, teaching and learning that are needed for family-centred care and provides the reader with a toolkit for use in practice.

The book has been designed to introduce the student nurse to family-centred care as a concept that underpins children's nursing and to enhance the practice of the qualified nurse. To facilitate student understanding of family-centred care, a variety of frameworks and definitions surrounding the concept are analysed and finally synthesized by the authors into an all encompassing definition and Practice Continuum in Part I of the book. Part II takes a theoretical and analytical approach to some of the current perspectives, issues and challenges impinging upon family-centred care. Thereafter, the main concerns of Part III are to address the skills needed to actually practice family-centred care and facilitate it becoming a living reality for children, families and nurses. The overall aim is to move the concept forward into the twenty-first century and prepare student nurses to meet the challenges of contemporary children's nursing.

LYNDA SMITH, VALERIE COLEMAN, MAUREEN BRADSHAW

Notes on the Contributors

Maureen Bradshaw is a Children's Nursing Lecturer at the University of Sheffield. Her interest in family-centred care has been shared in national and international publications and conferences.

Valerie Coleman is a Children's Nursing Lecturer at the University of Sheffield. She has published and presented nationally and internationally on the subject of family-centred care.

Sue Ford is Head of Education and Training at Sheffield Children's Hospital. Her interest in family-centred care stemmed largely from her previous role as a lecturer-practitioner in children's nursing in which she worked closely with pre-registration students.

Lynne Foxcroft is a Senior Lecturer in Law at the University of Huddersfield where she teaches medical law, criminal law and company law. She is a member of the ethics panel of the United Kingdom Central Council for Nursing, Midwifery and Health Visiting.

Gary Mountain is Senior Lecturer for Children's Nursing at the University of Huddersfield. His interests include methodological and ethical issues related to researching with children.

Lynda Smith is a Children's Nursing Lecturer at the University of Sheffield. She has worked extensively in the field of children's nursing practice both as a practitioner and lecturer.

Part I

THE CONCEPT OF FAMILY-CENTRED CARE AND THE SYNTHESIS OF A PRACTICE CONTINUUM

1

The Evolving Concept of Family-Centred Care

Valerie Coleman

Introduction

Family-centred care is a multifaceted concept that has evolved, over the past 50 years, to become a central tenet of children's nursing. Indeed Clayton (2000) suggests that culture in children's nursing has strengthened the concept to such an extent that nurses would not contemplate using an approach to childcare and nursing that did not advocate the involvement of families in care. However, in the plethora of literature that has been written about family-centred care, there appears to be no one single definition that clarifies the meaning of this concept, for use in practice. This may be attributed to family-centred care being a socially constructed concept, so that the definitions that are used to describe it are dependent upon the society from which they have emerged. Parenting and childhood as synonymous social constructs that are related to family-centred care will be explored later in Chapter 4.

Social evolvement of the concept has moved family-centred care progressively from relatively simple to more complex forms of association. It has moved from parental presence to parental involvement and participation, to partnership and eventually to the contemporary concept of family-centred care. The values of past societies, though, are still incorporated into future societies, according to Richman and Skidmore (2000). Hence, our contemporary social construction of family-centred care does reflect some values of previous societies in its philosophy. This further complicates the situation making it even more difficult to succinctly define the concept.

It is therefore not surprising that individual nurses, families and children have different understandings and perceptions, leading to nurses sometimes experiencing difficulties in implementing it in practice. The aim of this chapter is to explore the evolution of the social construction of family-centred care over the past 50 years and its importance and relevance in the twenty-first century. To be able to understand the social construction of family-centred care in the twenty-first century, it is helpful to have an historical perspective of its evolution. This exploration will influence its contemporary definition, which is to be suggested in Chapter 2.

Family-centred care: an evolving concept

The concept of family-centred care continues to evolve and expand, in Britain and other countries. A literature review suggests that its evolution has been influenced by several factors which could be grouped together under the following headings:

- Changing society, events and policies.
- Evolution of the theoretical underpinning of family-centred care.
- The responses of nurses and parents to family-centred care.

An exploration of each of these groups will now follow, including some references to how family-centred care has been socially constructed in its evolution.

Changing society, events and policies

The social world that is emphasized by social constructionists is one of multiple realities, according to Richman and Skidmore (2000). This means that the construct of family-centred care has undergone constant refinements of meaning, which are related to social actions and values. The accepted care settings for sick children have changed many times. 'The care of children in this country [Britain] has moved from care by the family in the home, to care by professionals in hospital and now care at home or in hospital by family and health care professionals' (Coyne, 1996, p. 739). The amount of involvement that families have had with their sick children in the hospital setting has also changed over time. Increasing professionalization of both medicine and nursing was initially responsible for families being excluded from having involvement in the care of their hospitalized child (Nethercott, 1993). It was believed that the presence of parents would inhibit care and visiting was restricted to effectively exclude parents from being with their child in hospital. Today's nurses are now expected to adopt an inclusion policy within which families are actively involved in care and are seen as the key stabilizing factor for the child (Campbell and Summersgill, 1993; Bradley, 1996). This illustrates that family-centred care as a social construct has undergone constant refinements in its meaning, dependent on the values and actions of the society within which that care has been practiced.

Key historical events in different societies, pre and post the 1950s, have influenced the evolution of family-centred care in Britain. The earlier events reflected a move away from sick children being cared for at home by their parents to routine admissions to hospital and the consequent exclusion of parents from care. Although interestingly, Dr George Armstrong in 1769 opened a dispensary (an outpatients department) in preference to a hospital, because if you separate a sick child from the parents 'you breaks its heart immediately' (cited by Miles 1986, p. 83). However, hospitals for sick children did begin to emerge in the nineteenth century and mother and child were inevitably separated.

This separation was in congruence with society at that time, with childhood being socially constructed to be barely distinguishable from adulthood. The emphasis was on physical care with little importance being attached to meeting the psychological needs of sick children in hospital. This was because of a major concern in the nineteenth and early-twentieth century with the prevalence of infectious diseases and other fatal illnesses. A hospital system was therefore created, for children, which was based upon asepsis and rigid routines to prevent cross infection (Darbyshire, 1993). The care of children in hospital, prior to the

1950s also reflected the behaviourist child-rearing ideologies of society. These advocated practices that meant adherence to routines that discouraged emotional interaction with children. The adoption of these ideologies further justified mechanistic and regimented care for children in hospital and also restricted parental visiting (Darbyshire, 1993).

The contemporary social construction of family-centred care began to emerge in the 1950s, though, as a result of the recognition of the emotional needs of children. This was brought about by the influential work of Bowlby (1953) on maternal deprivation in children's homes, and Robertson in 1958 studying the effects of maternal separation on hospitalized children (Robertson 1970). This work was reflected in the Platt Report (Ministry of Health, 1959), which made recommendations that recognized the importance of the hospitalized child's psychological welfare. One recommendation was that parents should be able to visit at any reasonable time of day or night. The National Association for the Welfare of Sick Children in Hospital (NAWCH) was formed in 1961, by parents, initially to advocate parental visiting. The Platt Report and the formation of NAWCH were influential events in the evolution of the social construction of family-centred care, with parental presence in hospital being valued by some elements of society at that time. However, the implementation of the Platt report was very slow according to Hall (1978), and unrestricted parental visiting was not an immediate reality. There was resistance from nurses and others who were not convinced that parental presence was a positive move.

Subsequent policy and organizations have continued to advocate, though, for the involvement of families in children's care both in hospital and home environments. The Court Report (Department of Health and Social Security, 1976) recognized that children have different needs from those of adults and that nurses and parents should work in partnership. The Children Act (Department of Health, 1989) emphasizes that parents are important to their children and have responsibilities towards them, suggesting that there is a requirement for nurses to adopt a family-centred approach to care. The *Welfare of Children and Young People in Hospital* (Department of Health, 1991) guidelines substantiate this, stating that 'a good quality service for children ... is child and family centred with children, their siblings and their parents or carers experiencing a "seamless web" of care and treatment, as they move through the constituent parts of the NHS'. NAWCH changed its name to Action for Sick Children in 1992, signifying a move towards more sick children being cared for at home by the family. The Audit Commission (1993) report on children's services in hospitals found that although the concept of family-centred care seemed to be accepted by children's nurses, its implementation could be improved in practice. *NHS: The Patient's Charter: Services for Children and Young People* (Department of Health, 1996) stated that families have a right and expectation to be involved in their child's care in both the hospital and community environments.

This exploration of changing society, events and policies, shows that the contemporary social construction of family-centred care for children is largely accepted in the twenty-first century, at least in the rhetoric. Targets issued by Action for Sick Children (1999) for the millennium, and standards for children in hospital drafted by the UK Committee for The United Nations Children Fund (UNICEF), Paediatric Nursing (1999/2000), do indeed advocate encouraging, supporting and empowering parents to care for their sick children.

Evolution of the theoretical underpinning of family-centred care

Bradley (1996) describes how in the early years of the evolution of family-centred care the knowledge that contributed towards socially constructing the concept came from disciplines external to nursing. Prior to the 1950s, the care of children in hospital was influenced by medical knowledge about infection control and strict child-rearing theories, which did not recognize the importance of a parental presence. Family-centred care theory which recognizes the importance of parental presence has been slowly developing since the 1950s, from a psychological perspective, strongly influenced by the work of Bowlby and Robertson. The earliest description of mother's presence emerged from doctors in 1958, describing projects where mothers were allowed to room-in with their children in specially designed units (Coyne, 1996). Doctors also wrote about the nurse's role in promoting the psychological care of children in hospital. 'Nurses should avoid doing everything themselves, but should take time to teach the mother how to care for her sick child' (Jolly, 1968, p. 17).

Some parents through their membership of NAWCH took the theory of family-centred care forwards not only by their advocacy of open parental visiting, which gradually became a reality, but also by monitoring and reporting on how the Platt Report's psychological recommendations were being implemented in practice throughout the country (Darbyshire, 1993).

However, Hall (1978) and Darbyshire (1994) both suggested that the Platt Report was too simplistic in not considering the sociological experiences of parents living in with their child in hospital and their relationships with nurses. In the early days of the theoretical development of family-centred care, the presence of parents with their sick child in hospital was not congruent with the social construction of children's nursing in hospital at that time. Richman and Skidmore (2000) describe how Marxist theory suggests that dominant groups have the power to impose their version of reality on others in society, by the very nature of the power they hold. The nurse's version of reality in hospital at this time seems to have been taken from a powerful medical profession, whose emphasis was on physical care. This version, it could be suggested, also gave nurses in turn some power over the parents, which they did not want to lose. Hence, parental presence often met with resistance and was not always actively encouraged.

An early nursing contribution to the theoretical evolution of the concept of family-centred care came from Hawthorne (1974). This study concluded that there were strong reasons for nurses to be taught about the emotional needs of children and for extending parental presence on the ward. Subsequently nurses were taught about the emotional needs of children in hospital, and by the 1980s the presence of parents with their children in hospital was accepted by many more nurses. The meaning of the social construction of family-centred care was refined at this time due to the social action that was being taken to develop the nurse's knowledge of children's emotional needs in hospital. This new knowledge perhaps empowered them to take some control and to change the accepted practices of children's nursing. Some nurses then began to undertake research studies for themselves about parental presence in hospital, and later on about the roles parents could undertake in their children's care.

These studies with their focus on roles suggested that family-centred care was constructed at this time to have a purely functional value with parents being expected to perform a range of different caring tasks for their hospitalized child. Darbyshire (1993) did identify that the roles undertaken by parents in hospital were considered in isolation from the role of children's nurses in these studies. This meant that the studies were potentially rather limited, because shared understandings or misunderstandings about nurses and parents roles were not captured in the findings.

Theory about parental roles was, nevertheless, translated into practice through the mechanism of separate care by parent units initially (Cleary *et al.*, 1986) and then by the development of care by parent units in general paediatric wards. These systems were meant to clarify for parents their caring roles and to free nurses 'to give ... greater attention to the sick children with complicated nursing needs' (Sainsbury *et al.*, 1986, p. 612). The social construct of family-centred care had been refined again and within this construct parents had moved from a passive presence to being allowed to take on a role in their child's care. Notably the roles that parents were 'allowed' to undertake were now more controlled by the nurse as opposed to the doctor, which was apparent in earlier constructions.

During the 1980s and the 1990s, nurses in Britain and other countries gradually accumulated a body of knowledge about the concept of family-centred care, created by nurses for nurses with the earlier influence of outside professionals diminishing (Bradley, 1996). Various nursing research studies have attempted to describe elements of the body of knowledge that explain family-centred care and to reflect the changing terminology associated with the concept in each new social construction. Studies have included parental involvement/parental participation (Dearmun, 1992; Neill, 1996) and partnership (Casey, 1995), negotiation of care roles (Callery and Smith, 1991) and empowerment of families (Marriott, 1990; Valentine, 1998). This literature has sought to explain the theoretical base of these elements and makes recommendations about how theory and practice could be developed. This accumulation of knowledge has led to a move away from special units to parental participation being encouraged wherever children are nursed. Fradd (1987) developed the concept further to include children and siblings as participants in care, clearly viewing parental participation as family participation.

Past research has tended to focus on family stress and dysfunction (Ahmann 1994), but it has now shifted to exploring family strengths and needs rather than weaknesses. This seems to reflect the contemporary values of society. Graves and Hayes (1996) and others have found that there is a lack of congruence, though, between how nurses and parents perceive parental needs. This suggests, 'that nurses need to learn from families, collectively and individually, what their needs are and ... to respond to what is learnt from families' (Ahmann, 1994, p. 113). Family-centred care in the twenty-first century requires nurses to work collaboratively with families. More research now needs to be undertaken to study the development of collaborative working relationships between nurses and families.

This exploration demonstrates how theory has evolved through different social constructions, from no parental presence, to parental presence, involvement, participation, partnership working and the empowerment of families. It could be concluded that one concept has replaced another. Cahill (1996), however, concluded in an analysis of parental participation that there is a hierarchical relationship between the concepts. However, because the values of past societies are incorporated into future societies all these concepts are still reflected in the contemporary practice of family-centred care, regardless of whether it is a hierarchical relationship or not.

Recent research studies (Baker, 1995; Bruce and Ritchie, 1997; Smith, 1998) have explored the application of this theory to practice and have found that despite family-centred care being taught in schools of nursing and nurses supporting the concept, there are difficulties transferring the theory into practice. Baker (1995) identified the main barriers to such transfer as being a lack of teacher support, role conflict, communication problems, power and control issues and communication problems. This was supported by Bruce and Ritchie (1997) who identified that more education was needed about practice activities involving negotiation and sharing information with families, as well as parental involvement in decision-making and planning of care. Bruce and Ritchie (1997) recommended that there was a need for skills development in areas of communication such as counselling, interviewing, interpersonal relationships and family dynamics.

Savage (2000) also identifies that in our nursing curricula there has been a greater emphasis on knowledge attainment rather than the development of necessary skills for the practice of family nursing. Skill development in nursing now needs to be fully addressed to enhance the delivery of family-centred care in practice. This is necessary to implement the contemporary theoretical social construction of family-centred care.

The responses of nurses and parents to family-centred care

The responses of both nurses and parents to the concept have contributed to its evolution, throughout different social constructions. The perspectives of both should be considered together, rather than in isolation. This is because it is important for nurses and parents to share their understandings of family centered care (Darbyshire, 1993). Parents and nurses are sometimes at odds with each other because they are attributing different attitudes and meanings to the concept.

Darbyshire (1993) describes a study undertaken by Meadows in 1964, post the Platt Report, which found that live-in parents became captive mothers akin to prisoners confined, not by bars, but by nursing expectations of their role. The parental role was one of passively sitting by the child's bedside with little or no participation in their child's care. Parents at this time wished to be present to meet their child's emotional needs, fearing that they would be upset if left alone in hospital. Parents perceived living on the ward to be a privilege, rather than an automatic right. This perception was congruent with society at this time, which was not so focused on the rights of the individual, as is the contemporary society of the twenty-first century.

Nurses also appeared to be wary of parents, tolerating their presence, rather than actively encouraging it (Darbyshire, 1993). In Hawthorne's (1974) study it was found that only one of nine wards actually encouraged mothers to stay, despite 84 per cent of interviewed nurses denying that mothers got in the way of nurses.

Nurses gradually came to accept the presence of parents on the ward, allowing them to undertake some aspects of their child's care. Darbyshire (1993) found that in subsequent studies parents were comfortable with carrying out non-technical aspects of care related to giving emotional support, accompanying children for tests and doing usual childcare practices. The parents were less sure about their ability to perform more technical nursing care; they were anxious about making a mistake and were unwilling to upset the hospital routine by getting in the way. Initially nurses were also reluctant to release the technical tasks to parents. However, as more children have survived with conditions which previously would have led to short life expectancies, parents have had to take on these nursing tasks and the social construction of family-centred care has evolved to encompass this development.

Theoretically, the concept has evolved to be about working in partnership with parents, but in practice there is evidence that nurses do not always respond to parents as equal partners in care planning and decision-making processes, 'paying lip service to a notion of partnership based on equality and mutual respect' (Dearmun, 1992, p. 17). This may be because nurses have a tendency to focus on enabling parents to give direct care to their children, because of the commonly held view of parents as 'essentially being of functional value' (Darbyshire, 1993, p. 1678). Nurses should also be finding out what parental participation means for individual families and developing professional relationships to help them with the process, so that partnership working becomes a reality in practice.

Ahmann (1994) and Baker (1995) suggest that, traditionally, nurses have been in control and have held the power when working with families. It has already been identified that nurses in the past have been reluctant to relinquish this power to children and families to enable them to be true partners in care. Campbell and Summersgill (1993) stated that initially nurses did not act upon separation work (Bowlby, 1953; Robertson, 1970) because of a paternalistic working environment and the limited extent of their own empowerment to make changes in the system of healthcare delivery. It can be argued that many nurses are still not empowered, as demonstrated in Baker's (1995) study. Hence, it is unlikely that these nurses will be negotiating care with families, teaching them to give care and empowering them to be in control by participating in decision-making about their child's care.

It has become apparent in the literature that, 'discontinuity can arise between the perspectives of family and professionals regarding their respective roles in providing care for children in hospital' (Savage, 2000, p. 34). Nurses sometimes take it for granted that parents want more involvement in their child's care, whereas parents may actually want less involvement, especially in the area of clinical and technical procedures which some parents can find distressing (Coyne, 1995; Neill, 1996). Darbyshire (1994) also found that caring for a sick child in public can be extremely stressful for parents and it certainly will be if reluctant parents feel obliged to be involved in care without appropriate preparation. Conversely, Savage (2000) suggests that some nurses' expectations of parents assuming a passive role conflicts with the parents' expectations of themselves becoming increasingly involved in their child's care in hospital. These different perceptions can be disempowering to families and emphasize the power and control of nurses.

Recent nursing research suggests that the concept of family-centred care has evolved to mean more than mechanistic roles. Hutchfield (1999) found that the key elements of the contemporary social construction were seen to be respect for parents, a concern for family well-being, collaborative working in the form of partnership, shared decision-making and effective communication, as well as involving parents in the care of their child. However, these views are not always reflected in nursing practice (Baker, 1995; Bruce and Ritchie, 1997; Bridgman, 1999). This may be because nurses are reluctant to relinquish their power, but it could also be due to a lack of resources to support family-centred care in practice, notably sufficient time to communicate, which is a necessary precursor of such care (Hutchfield, 1999). Nurses need to overcome these barriers to be able to work collaboratively with children and families in the practice of family-centred care in the twenty-first century.

Advancing contemporary nursing practice in the twenty-first century

Our ever-changing society drives the healthcare system which is also influenced and driven from without by international forces such as the UNICEF Child Friendly Hospitals Initiative (Paediatric Nursing, 1999/2000), and from within by its own policy-makers and standard-setters, for example the Department of Health's (1996) *NHS: The Patient's Charter: Services for Children and Young People.* These current standards now require healthcare workers to facilitate a family-centred approach to care, but what has not yet been determined is the criteria that will be used to measure it. Children's nurses in collaboration with parents, however, are in a prime position to drive and influence the achieving of family-centred care standards. Issues surrounding some of the real and perceived barriers to this will be explored in later chapters.

If family-centred care has been evolving in order to try and maintain some congruence with the ever-changing society over the last 50 years, then the next question is how can we continue to ensure that the evolution of the concept remains dynamic in order to sustain its relevance for children and their families in the twenty-first century? It must be research that continues to drive this evolution in order to ensure that the practice of family-centred care becomes increasingly evidence-based. Savage (2000) suggests that going into hospital is no longer such a hazard as it once was for children, and anxieties about the detrimental effects of hospitalization have now passed. This highlights that there are more contemporary issues that need to be addressed in research.

Family-centred care was initially socially constructed in acute settings in the UK. Conversely, in North America it was constructed in social settings within which there were children with special needs. There has been a tendency to utilize the concept in other settings without always acknowledging that the needs of children and families may differ. Further evolution of the concept should ensure that a more flexible approach is used to ensure it is meeting the needs of the client group in each individual setting.

Also, the profile of the acutely-ill child in hospital has changed according to Rennick (1995). This signifies that the family-centred care concept needs to be socially reconstructed to respond to this change. Previously, children who were hospitalized had acute illnesses that were of relatively short durations and recovery soon took place. Early research pertinent to family-centred care was conducted with the aforementioned children and their families. The situation is different now because children with an acute illness are often much sicker and families are forced to endure increasingly difficult situations with uncertain outcomes for longer periods of time (Rennick, 1995). The focus of research and practice needs to change to studying family processes and interactions, instead of concentrating on the individual child or parent, suggests Rennick (1995). This would seem an appropriate change and there is already some evidence of the concept evolving to focus more on the needs of the whole family. This is a development that nurses need to pursue to ensure that children and families with an acute illness today are being supported adequately during difficult times.

Many other children experience only short stays in hospital and the numbers that are admitted as day cases have increased. This means that there are more sick children who need continuing care currently being looked after at home by their families, than in previous years. Therefore family-centred care as a social construction seems to have evolved full circle back into the community setting. However, society and illness have both changed and the construct in the twenty-first century in the community is different from that prior to the opening of children's hospitals in the nineteenth century.

Children and their families at home in the community are often experts regarding their own situation and condition. Savage (2000) discusses the concept of discontinuity from differing perspectives, including discontinuity when children with a chronic illness are admitted to hospital. It is suggested that family care is discontinued to some extent on hospitalization because nurses take over the child's care without always recognizing the expertise of the family. The family then have to resume care when the child is discharged home, which potentially leads to further discontinuity of care. Recent evolvement of the concept has included attempts to ensure that there is a seamless web of family-centred care at the interface between hospital and community, to avoid this discontinuity. This signifies a need for partnerships with families and collaborative working.

To enable this to happen successfully there seems to be a need to address the education of nurses. There is evidence (Baker, 1995, and Bruce and Ritchie, 1997) that nurses have a good understanding and knowledge base about family-centred care as a theoretical concept. However, evidence from the same studies found that nurses had difficulties in translating this theoretical knowledge into practice for various reasons. As previously highlighted, Bruce and Ritchie (1997) found in their study that nurses reported a lack of adequate education in relation to understanding and practicing the concept, which indicates a need for nurses to be enabled to develop the skills of empowerment, negotiation and teaching through the process of nurse education.

Summary

The social construct of family-centred care has evolved, reflecting many changes in our society. Policy has advocated the need for such care, although its implementation in practice has often been slow. The theoretical underpinning of family-centred care has gradually developed, with the focus of studies gradually changing. Initially the focus was on the effects of separating mother and child, but nowadays studies are increasingly exploring family processes. Knowledge was developed in the early days by sources external to nursing, but in time nurses began to undertake research about family-centred care for themselves. Nurses and parents do not always share the same perceptions about such care, but their responses to it have helped with ongoing construction and refinement of the meaning of the construct.

Family-centred care remains a significant concept for the twenty-first century. To make it a reality in practice, in all settings, we need to focus on partnerships and collaborative working with families, together with the development of the appropriate skills in practitioners to facilitate this. The Practice Continuum, in Chapter 2, is a framework that has the potential to enable nurses to implement contemporary social constructions of family-centred care in both hospital and community settings.

References

Action for Sick Children (1999) *Ten Targets for the Millennium* (London: Action for Sick Children).

Ahmann, E. (1994) 'Family-Centred Care: Shifting Orientation', *Pediatric Nursing*, March–April, 20(2), pp. 113–6.

Audit Commission (1993) *Children First: A Study of Hospital Services* (London: HMSO).

Baker, S. (1995) 'Family Centred Care: A Theory Practice Dilemma', *Paediatric Nursing,* July, 7(6), pp. 17–20

Bowlby, J. (1953) *Child Care and the Growth of Love* (Harmondsworth: Penguin).

Bradley, S. (1996) 'Processes in the Creation and Diffusion of Nursing Knowledge: An Examination of the Developing Concept of Family Centred Care', *Journal of Advanced Nursing,* 23, pp. 722–7.

Bridgman, J. (1999) 'How do Nurses Learn about Family-Centred Care?' *Paediatric Nursing,* May, 11(4), pp. 26–9.

Bruce, B. and Ritchie, J. (1997) 'Nurses' Practices and Perceptions of Family Centred Care', *Journal of Pediatric Nursing,* August, 12(4), pp. 214–22.

Callery, P. and Smith, L. (1991) 'A Study of Role Negotiation Between Nurses and the Parents of Hospitalised Children', *Journal of Advanced Nursing,* 16, pp. 772–81.

Cahill, J. (1996) 'Patient Participation: A Concept Analysis', *Journal of Advanced Nursing,* 24, pp. 561–71.

Campbell, S. and Summersgill, P. (1993) 'Keeping it in the Family: Defining and Developing Family Centred Care', *Child Health,* June/July, pp. 17–20.

Casey, A. (1995) 'Partnership Nursing: Influences on Involvement of Informal Carers', *Journal of Advanced Nursing,* 22, pp. 1058–62.

Clayton, M. (2000) 'Health and Social Policy: Influences on Family Centred Care', *Paediatric Nursing,* October, 12(8), pp. 31–3.

Cleary, J., Gray, O., Hall, D., Rowlandson, D. and Sainsbury, C. (1986) 'Parental Involvement in the Lives of Children in Hospital', *Archives of Disease in Childhood,* 61(8), pp. 779–87.

Coyne, I. (1995) 'Parental Participation in Care: A Critical Review of the Literature', *Journal of Advanced Nursing,* 21, pp. 716–22.

Coyne, I. (1996) 'Parent Participation: A Concept Analysis', *Journal of Advanced Nursing,* 723, pp. 733–40.

Darbyshire, P. (1993) 'Parents, Nurses and Paediatric Nursing: A Critical Review', *Journal of Advanced Nursing,* 18, pp. 1670–180.

Darbyshire, P. (1994) *Living with a Sick Child in Hospital: The experiences of parents and nurses* (London: Chapman & Hall).

Dearmun, A. (1992) 'Perceptions of Parental Participation', *Paediatric Nursing,* September, 4(7), pp. 6–9.

Department of Health and Social Security (1976) *Fit for the Future: The Court Report* (London: HMSO).

Department of Health (1989) *An Introduction to The Children Act 1989* (London: HMSO).

Department of Health (1991) *Welfare of Children and Young People in Hospital* (London: HMSO).

Department of Health (1996) *NHS: The Patient's Charter: Services for Children and Young People* (London: HMSO).

Fradd, E. (1987) 'A Child Alone', *Nursing Times,* 83(42), pp. 16–7.

Graves, C. and Hayes, V. (1996) 'Do Nurses and Parents of Children with Chronic Conditions Agree on Parental Needs?' *Journal of Pediatric Nursing,* 11(5), pp. 288–99.

Hall, D. (1978) 'Bedside Blues: the Impact of Social Research on the Hospital Treatment of Sick Children', *Journal of Advanced Nursing,* 3, pp. 25–37.

Hawthorne, P. (1974) *Nurse – I Want My Mummy* (London: Royal College of Nursing).

Hutchfield, K. (1999) 'Family Centred Care: A Concept Analysis', *Journal of Advanced Nursing,* 29(5), pp. 1178–87.

Jolly, H. (1968) *Diseases of Children,* 2nd edn (Oxford: Blackwell Scientific Publications).

Kawik, L. (1996) 'Nurses Attitudes and Perceptions of Parental Participation', *British Journal of Nursing,* 5(7), pp. 430–4.

Marriott, S. (1990) 'Parent Power', *Nursing Times,* 86(34), pp. 65.

Miles, I. (1986) 'The Emergence of Sick Children's Nursing Part 1. Sick Children's Nursing before the Turn of the Century', *Nurse Education Today,* 6, pp. 82–7.

Ministry of Health and Central Health Services Council (1959) *The Welfare of Children in Hospital, Platt Report* (London: HMSO).

Neill, S. (1996) 'Parent Participation 2: Findings and their Implications for Practice', *British Journal of Nursing,* 5(2), pp. 110–7.

Nethercott, S. (1993) 'Family Centred Care: A Concept Analysis', *Professional Nurse,* September, pp. 794–7.

Paediatric Nursing (1999/2000) 'Global Millennium Targets: UNICEF Child Friendly Hospital Initiative', *Paediatric Nursing,* December/January, 11(10), pp. 7–8.

Rennick, J. (1995) 'The Changing Profile of Acute Childhood Illness: A Need for the Development of Family Nursing Knowledge', *Journal of Advanced Nursing,* 22(2), pp. 258–66.

Richman, J. and Skidmore, D. (2000) 'Health Implications of Modern Childhood', *Journal of Child Health Care,* 4(3), Autumn, pp. 106–10.

Robertson, J. (1970) *Young Children in Hospital,* 2nd edn (London: Tavistock Publications).

Sainsbury, C. P. Q., Gray, O. P., Cleary, J., Davies, M. M. and Rowlandson, P. H. (1986) 'Care by Parents of their Children in Hospital', *Archives of Disease in Childhood,* 61, pp. 612–5.

Savage, E. (2000) 'Family Nursing: Minimising Discontinuity for Hospitalised Children and their Families', *Paediatric Nursing,* March, 12(2), pp. 33–7.

Smith, L. (1998) 'Student Nurses' Experiences of Family Centred Care and their Relationship to Theory Practice Issues', unpublished Masters dissertation: University of Sheffield.

Valentine, F. (1998) 'Empowerment: Family Centred Care', *Paediatric Nursing,* February, 10(1), pp. 24–7.

2

Family-Centred Care: A Practice Continuum

Lynda Smith, Valerie Coleman and Maureen Bradshaw

Introduction

The evolving concept of family-centred care has the potential to promote the health of children and families in the twenty-first century, and the integration of the concept into practice should reflect a contemporary definition of such care. 'The work of caring for parents [though] has been found to be ad hoc and unpredictable' (Callery, 1997, p. 992), causing difficulties for both nurses and parents. In addition to developing the appropriate skills for practice, nurses also need to re-examine the approaches that they use to implement the concept in practice:

> Improving practices with families of paediatric patients is most likely to occur when nurses and other health care professionals, fully understand the characteristics and consequences of using different approaches in their work. (Dunst and Trivette, 1996, p. 334)

Several definitions and theoretical frameworks have been offered to explain the elements of family-centred care, and are reflected in the different approaches used by nurses in their implementation of the concept. Some of these will be explored in this chapter, which will culminate in a contemporary definition of the concept and our synthesis of a continuum for its practice.

19

Finally, scenarios will be used to illustrate the use of the continuum in a variety of situations, for individual families.

Defining family-centred care

Family-centred care is used as an all-embracing term to describe a concept with many different attributes, and to some extent this has contributed to some of the confusion that surrounds its application in practice. Thus we have terms such as parental involvement, parental participation, care by parents, family nursing and partnership nursing. What do these terms mean, in what ways are they describing the same thing or something different? How are these terms linked and are they all referring to family-centred care or a facet of such care? In order to answer these questions it is necessary to define some of the terms in common usage and clarify their meaning in relation to the concept.

Family-centred care is underpinned by professionals recognizing the central role of the family in the child's life. The family is actively involved in care to the extent they choose, which requires a collaborative partnership with the family (Ahmann, 1998). Theoretical frameworks that have developed the basic concept will be explored in more detail later in the chapter, including Shelton and Smith Stepanek's (1995) framework of family-centred care, Nethercott's (1993) components of family-centred care and Hutchfield's (1999) hierarchy of family-centred care.

Parental involvement sometimes appears in the literature as synonymous with the term parent participation (Darbyshire, 1994). Parental involvement in care is also seen as a precursor to family-centred care in so far as parents are enabled to be with their child at all times, involve themselves in basic care and to an extent decision-making, but the nurse remains in control of the family's involvement (Nethercott, 1993).

Parent participation in care has been the subject of research (Dearmun, 1992; Evans, 1994; Kawik, 1996; Neill, 1996), but largely from the perspective of parent and nurse perceptions of the reality of the concept in practice. No clear consensus appears concerning the meaning of parent participation. Neill (1996) utilized a definition that encompassed parents being involved in decision-making, delivery of care or just being consulted on their child's care, with parents having the ability to choose the level of participation, which necessitated negotiation between parents and professionals.

Nethercott (1993) distinguishes between the two terms in so far as parent participation incorporates the features of parental involvement but parents are seen more as partners in care, able also to take on more complex tasks. The distinction is also made between expectation and negotiation, with the assumption being that parents willingly undertake aspects of care.

Care by Parent describes specific units where parents have responsibility for providing their child's daily care with support from nurses. An example of this is provided by Sainsbury *et al.* (1986), who defined this system as one where the parent's role is clarified, giving active participation and responsibility for their child's recovery. This released nurses from some of their nursing procedures enabling them to undertake the 'superior role' of advising and counselling. Thus the nurse is seen as the expert in the child's care and again certain tasks are delegated to parents.

Family nursing is an approach to care based on the belief that the family is integral to the child, and it therefore involves nurses perceiving the care of families as part of their role (Savage, 2000). According to Wright and Leahey (1994), cited by Savage (2000), this can be approached in three different ways:

- *Individual as focus*: In this approach nursing focuses on the individual and the family are in the background. The family is involved in the child's care and provides support to their child supported by the nurse as needed. This approach clearly links to the earlier definition of parental involvement.
- *Family as focus*: In this approach the family is the client and therefore nursing care focuses on every individual. Thus a resident parent's needs, for example, are part of the care provided.
- *Family as unit of care or family systems nursing*: This approach focuses on the family as a whole simultaneously. Thus parents may be involved in the care of their child, but need the support of the nurse at the same time.

This latter approach links with the *Partnership* model developed by Casey (1988), in which parent participation is viewed in terms of partnership with parents. The role of parents in caring for their child is fully acknowledged to the extent that children are best cared for by their parents with varying amounts of help from the healthcare professional as necessary. The emphasis is the family as the focus of care providing that care with assistance from the nurse, hence the link with the family as the unit of care.

Family-centred-care can be seen as a composite of these different terms as they have evolved over time. They all acknowledge the family's role in the care of their child but to varying and differing extents. Parental involvement and parental participation tend to be nurse-led in orientation, while partnership nursing infers equality between nurse and family in the caring process. At the far end of the spectrum care may be led by parents, experts in all aspects of the care of their child, and the nurse's role in this instance is more consultative.

The level of family-centred care subscribed to by parents is underpinned by specific attributes that support the concept, namely collaboration, negotiation, empowerment, support through teaching and advocacy and sharing in an open and honest environment. The extent to which these attributes are utilized depends on the skill of the nurse in facilitating them and the wishes of the parent in relation to the extent to which they wish to lead or be led in the care of their child. Ultimately all of the terms described, with their associated attributes, offer different dimensions of family-centred care, each in their own way relevant and providing an opportunity for families to be involved in the care of their child, preferably to an extent of their choosing.

An overarching contemporary definition of family-centred care could therefore be seen as:

The professional support of the child and family through a process of involvement, participation and partnership underpinned by empowerment and negotiation.

How this is then interpreted in practice is underpinned and supported by frameworks for family-centred care and models for paediatric practice.

Theoretical frameworks

Theoretical frameworks can be explained using the following headings:

- A comparison of functional and holistic frameworks for family-centred care.
- Communication frameworks.
- Hierarchical frameworks.

A comparison of functional and holistic frameworks for family-centred care

Hutchfield (1999) identifies that two views of family-centred care have emerged. One view is functional and lacks collaboration, 'with the nurse taking the role of gatekeeper and dominant player, deciding what care the parent can participate in' (Hutchfield 1999, p. 1181), which is reflected in approaches to family-centred care that allow parents to perform tasks, to enable them to feel useful (Darbyshire, 1993), and uses checklists of childcare activities that mothers are prepared to do (Coyne, 1995). Roles are also allocated to parents, when the functional, nurse-led approach is used, such as 'vigilant parent or nurturer-comforter' (Snowden and Gottlieb, 1989, cited by Coyne, 1995, p. 717).

Nethercott (1993) identified seven key critical components of family-centred care (Table 2.1). Although some of the components do recognise the importance of viewing the family in context, 'the majority of the other components appear to focus on supporting the functional role of the family' (Hutchfield, 1999, p. 1180). The functional view is reflected in components such as the performance of usual childcare practices, which unless detrimental to the child's well-being should be continued in hospital, and families who want to may be involved in technical aspects of care (Nethercott, 1993). These critical components do seem to describe a functional approach to family-centred care.

Darbyshire (1993) suggests that when parents are understood as being of essentially functional value, they become problems or resources to be effectively used by nurses. This results in 'socially

Table 2.1   A summary of the critical components for family-centred care identified by Nethercott (1993)

- The family must be viewed in its normal context
- The roles of individual family members must be evaluated to maximize their individual roles in the provision of care for their child
- Specific information about the child's illness should be given to the family to enable them to participate in decision-making
- The prime caregiver should be involved in care planning
- Family involvement in technical aspects of care should be dependant on their ability and willingness to participate
- The family should continue with their usual provision of childcare in hospital, providing it is not detrimental to the child's condition
- The family should be evaluated to determine their needs for support following the discharge or death of the child

---

engineered solutions being sought rather than exploring the meaning of parental participation' (Darbyshire, 1993, p. 1678), which is a feature more characteristic of a holistic approach to family-centred care. The power remains with the nurse in the role of the aforementioned gatekeeper and families may be actually disempowered by the use of a functional approach.

Conversely, the holistic view identified by Hutchfield (1999) is more likely to be empowering to children and families. It 'represents a description of family centred care, which is grounded in respect for and cooperation with the family' (Hutchfield, 1999, p. 1181). The nurse acts as an equal partner and a facilitator of care when this approach is used. It is an approach that 'requires nurses to shift from a professionally centred view of health care to a collaborative model that recognises the family as central in a child's life' (Ahmann, 1994, p. 113). The values and priorities of the families are viewed as central to the care that is planned for the child. This view of family-centred care had its origins within the framework of elements identified in 1987 by Shelton *et al.* in the USA (Shelton and Smith Stepanek, 1995). A revision of this framework in 1994 changed the presentation order of the elements (Table 2.2), with the first element now recognizing that the family are the constant in the child's life, and the following elements building up on each other, linked together by a strong thread of communication.

This framework was developed for children and families with special needs, which may explain why it differs from the more

Table 2.2 A summary of the key elements of family-centred care identified by Shelton and Smith Stepanek (1995)

- Values the family as the constant in the child's life and recognizes that the supportive services will fluctuate
- Family and professionals work together in collaboration, at all levels of care
- Complete and unbiased information is exchanged between the family and professionals
- Recognizes and responds to the cultural diversity within and between families
- Meets the diverse needs of families and respects different ways of coping
- Promotes family-to-family support and networking
- Provides flexible, accessible, comprehensive services that are responsive to diverse family needs
- Accepts that families are families and children are children first and foremost, possessing a wide range of strengths and concerns and the child's health may not always be the only family priority
- Communication is the thread that weaves these inter-related elements together

Together these elements of family-centred care result in policies and practices that recognize the pivotal role of the family in their child's care

functional one offered by Nethercott (1993). In Britain, the concept of family-centred care initially developed as a functional approach within acute care settings for children.

The Shelton *et al.* framework of family-centred care from 1987 and its subsequent revisions all promote the use of nursing strategies that include 'recognizing and accepting diverse styles of family coping, helping families recognize their strengths and methods of coping, reassuring parents regarding their essential role and facilitating family involvement and care giving' (Ahmann, 1994, p. 113). The functional approach is characterized by a tendency to identify family problems and weaknesses. Conversely, the holistic approach explores families' strengths and builds on these in the care of the child. By enabling the family to recognize their own strengths, it facilitates them taking some control over their situation, and family-centred care may eventually become parent-led. The aforementioned functional approach seems to limit the ability of the family to gain any control over their situation (Baker, 1995). The holistic approach also identifies the importance of exchanging complete and unbiased information with families (Shelton and Smith Stepanek, 1995). This facilitates nurses learning from parents about the child and family, which is a necessary prerequisite of working in equal partnership.

This comparison between the functional and holistic views of family-centred care demonstrates that there are two approaches that could be used to implement the philosophy of such care that have fundamentally different underlying philosophies. It could be suggested that communication is a common feature of both views, but the approaches used differ because the holistic view is more about mutuality and open communication than the functional view. The adoption of a functional approach in practice does not prevent nurses using communication skills such as negotiation. However, when a functional approach is used there is likely to be a lack of mutuality between nurses and families, because the focus will be on the functional role of parents rather than family empowerment. Callery and Smith (1991) seemed to find evidence of this in a study on negotiation. Some nurses negotiated with parents with a rigid set of expectations, whilst other nurses had less rigid expectations about parents in the negotiation process. It could be suggested the nurses with the less rigid expectations were pursuing a holistic approach to family-centred care, and their colleagues a functional approach. Partnerships involve 'the sharing of mutually agreed roles between the nurse and patient, communicating and listening to parents and supporting parents in their child's care' (Valentine, 1998, p. 26).

Communication frameworks

Ahmann (1994) proposes that the use of communication models can contribute to the development of true collaborative parent–nurse partnerships, which do not happen too easily for most nurses, other professionals or parents. 'Nurses need to learn how to restructure communication with parents so that it becomes more collaborative' (Ahmann, 1994, p. 115).

Casey (1995) developed a framework to describe the effect of communication and nursing style on family involvement in care of children in hospital. Using this framework some practitioners are nurse-centred and are authoritative and controlling in their communications with families. They do assess parental wishes and allow them to become involved in care, but it is on the nurse's terms and centres on permission being granted. Other nurse-centred practitioners, according to Casey (1995), are non-communicating and continue the traditional practice of excluding parents from their child's care, making all kinds of assumptions about families needs, wishes and abilities. Conversely other person-centred nurses do communicate and negotiate with parents, and Casey (1995) suggests that these are skilled paediatric nurses who are willing to share their knowledge and expertise and to listen to families. Perhaps these skilled nurses are ones that in the terms of Ahmann (1994) have restructured their communication skills to become collaborative in working with children and families.

This would certainly seem to be required for family-centred care; otherwise

> without good communication assumptions are made by parents too, about what constitutes nursing and what is expected of them in hospital. Misunderstanding and conflict arise if mutual expectations and assumptions are not explicitly addressed. (Casey, 1995, p. 1061).

Two communication models that may assist the restructuring process are the 1983 LEARN framework for communication by Berlin and Fowkes, and the 1988 Nursing Mutual Participation Model of care by Curley both cited by Ahmann (1994). These are suggested to be models that provide a shift from the unidirectional way in which many nurses have interacted with parents.

The LEARN Model is strongly focused on the need for families and nurses to listen carefully to each other and to acknowledge differences and similarities in their individual perceptions of problems, prior to negotiating about the child's care (the acronym LEARN represents L = listen, to families perceptions, E = explain your perception as the nurse, A = acknowledge and discuss differences and similarities, R = recommend treatment, N = negotiate agreement). The Nursing Mutual Participation Model is about searching by the use of open-ended questions in a caring atmosphere for what the child and family may feel is most useful for them to do in respect of participation in care, because 'the professional alone cannot know what is best for the child' (Ahmann, 1994, p. 115).

To be able to implement the holistic view of family-centred care, some model of communication needs to be incorporated into nursing practice. In reality, practice may be constrained by the nursing models that are used to organize care. Many of them focus on the individual patient, rather than the family, and collaborative partnerships are not part of the philosophies underpinning these models. Models for children's nursing have been developed, notably the Partnership Model by Casey and Mobbs (1988), which could facilitate the use of some of the aforementioned communication strategies for collaborative partnership working. 'The Partnership Model of paediatric nursing evolved as a description of nursing practice – serving as a guide to developing the nursing process in a more suitable way for children's nursing' (Casey and Mobbs, 1988, p. 68). It evolved to acknowledge the concept of family-centred care and was

> based on a recognition of and respect for a family's expertise in the care of their child ... if a family member is present or the child themselves wishes to be self caring, a process of negotiation is entered into, with the nurse providing continuous support and teaching to enable the family to make informed decisions about care and their part in it. (Casey, 1995, p. 1059)

It is suggested, though, by Coyne (1996) that despite its title the partnership model contradicts the concept of partnership because it implies that the nurse is only concerned with the family as carers of the child and the roles that they can assume in care. A collaborative partnership is concerned more with communication and developing a relationship between the nurse and family than this model suggests, according to Coyne (1996). Conversely, Savage (2000) views the Partnership Model as very conducive to family systems nursing, which encompasses a holistic approach that views the whole family as a unit of care. Savage (2000) interprets the Partnership Model as being one that is concerned with the structure of the family, the relationships within it and forces affecting it. These two different interpretations of the same model demonstrates that conceptual models can be implemented in different ways by practitioners and, in effect, this particular model could be utilized both within a functional approach and a holistic one to family-centred care. It is acknowledged, though, that this concept continues to evolve and hence nursing models can be interpreted differently over time. Another argument could be that because nurses may lack the skills of negotiation, empowerment and teaching, there is a tendency to use conceptual models functionally rather than holistically. There is evidence from several studies that nurses understand the concept of family-centred, but do not use their skills to put it into practice (Baker, 1995; Bruce and Ritchie, 1997).

Hierarchical frameworks

Several reasons have been given to explain why the practice of family-centred care has lagged behind a conceptual acceptance of the philosophy, according to Ahmann (1994). One reason is that some confusion appears to exist about the different approaches that can be used in the care of families in practice. There seems to have been a move from parental involvement to parental participation to partnership working, and finally to family-centred care. In other words, one concept replacing another in each different social construction, or alternatively as suggested by Cahill (1996) there is a hierarchical relationship between the concepts. It does appear that in both the functional and holistic approaches, involvement, participation and partnership are all practiced under the nomenclature of family-centred care. In reality though, Hutchfield (1999) suggests these concepts could be viewed as precursors and family-centred care in its fullest sense is only implemented in some cases. Hutchfield (1999) offers a hierarchical framework for the practice of family-centred care which has four levels proceeding from involvement at the lowest level, through to participation, partnership and finally family-centred care at the highest level of the hierarchy. The differences between the levels are clearly explained under the following headings: type of relationship; beliefs about the parents and family; characteristics of the level of care; communication required; and identification of both parental and nursing roles at individual levels.

A strength of this framework is that it recognizes that families want to participate in the care of their children in hospital at a level of their own choosing. This is important because evidence suggests that different parents desire differing levels of participation (Coyne, 1995, p. 718). When attempts are made to apply family-centred care at an inappropriate level for a family it 'creates the potential for the development of unnecessary stress for children, families and professionals' (Hutchfield, 1999, p. 1186). Nurses through accurate assessment and negotiation with children and families could use Hutchfield's (1999) hierarchical framework to identify the level of care that an individual family may wish to engage in, and then prepare the family for participation at that desired level. The framework provides a clear indication of the differences between the levels, together with the implications of this for the practice of family-centred care.

Negatively, there is the potential for nurses to only use this hierarchical framework to designate the levels of care for individual families and not to find out about the experiences of parents living in hospital with a sick child as advocated by Darbyshire (1994). This is because a forward linear movement through predictable stages 'sits comfortably with Western and traditional scientific understanding' (Darbyshire, 1994, p. 14). The framework seems to suggest that movement is forward up the hierarchy and it does not appear to reflect that the level of care, which families may wish to give to their children, can vary over time.

Family-centred care: a Practice Continuum

Having analysed the theoretical frameworks in use and identified the evolving concept of family-centred care and the interrelationship of the different terms and attributes that underpin it, it is clear that there is the potential for family-centred care to operate at different levels. This would or could be in response to differing parental needs and differing abilities on the part of nurses to fully negotiate and be partners in care.

Thus, rather than offer a hierarchical approach to family-centred care, where such care is seen as utopia with the ultimate achievement being parent-led care, it can be viewed alternatively as a Practice Continuum where parents choose where they wish to be on the continuum. This may also vary as circumstances change during the course of their child's care. In viewing family-centred care as a Practice Continuum it is possible to incorporate all the elements of the various theoretical frameworks. Thus a functional approach would suit parental participation and parental involvement which is still essentially nurse-led, but where parents do feel involved in the care of their child. Shelton and Smith Stepanek's (1995) holistic framework would sit comfortably with the partnership approach that strives towards equality in the relationship.

Communication frameworks facilitate the development of those skills in nurses which support the key attributes of collaboration and negotiation which are present throughout the continuum but especially so in the partnership approach. If as the literature would suggest (Baker, 1995; Bruce and Ritchie, 1997) nurses understand the concept of family-centred care but do not use their skills to put it into practice, then utilizing a communication framework may well support nurses putting theory into practice.

The hierarchical framework proposed by Hutchfield (1999) clearly identifies the different dimensions within family-centred care, but in terms of levels, with the final level to be achieved being family-centred care. Whilst this is well-elucidated and logical in its development, the inference is that such care would only be achievable for a small group, given the descriptors attributed to it. Yet family-centred care is acknowledged throughout children's nursing in a much broader way and to say that only those parents with extensive knowledge of their child's illness and treatment, who are experts in all aspects of the care of their child, are party to family-centred care in its fullest sense is to demean the role of parents and nurses working to different goals in the support of the child and family.

Whilst acknowledging the significance of Hutchfield's work in this area, particularly in the descriptions of the different facets of parental participation, parental involvement and partnership, it seems more relevant to the concept of family-centred care to see all these terms as differing dimensions of the concept. Clarification of the nature of both parents and nurses involvement in facilitating such care is imperative if the concept is to move forward and avoid the difficulties experienced so far in its interpretation and operationalization in practice. The Practice Continuum offers a more readily understood view of family-centred care for practitioners, who could feel they were operationalizing care within a particular dimension of the Practice Continuum.

Professionally, family-centred care is the stated philosophy for children's nurses and underpins the philosophy of paediatric units throughout the country, and is thus at the heart of children's nursing practice. Parents are familiar with the term without being concerned with the specifics of the level they are involved at, provided they have the opportunity to participate to the extent they wish and not the extent they are allowed.

By facilitating a clearer understanding of the terms within the overall concept, some of the confusion can be alleviated and parents and nurses can mutually determine their contribution to family-centred care without some of the pressures experienced by both groups previously. For various reasons it may only be possible to facilitate nurse-led involvement or participation in care, but in other circumstances a more parent-led approach may ensue.

Thus family-centred care is seen as the range of parental input varying from being nurse-led, to sharing equal status and being parent-led. There is no ultimate goal to be achieved and where the nurse or parent is located on the Practice Continuum may vary with each admission, contact or according to the ability of the nurse or parent to facilitate that part of the Continuum. Where problems may occur is if there is an expectation—experience mismatch between the parents and the nurse. Open communication is therefore essential to the facilitation of the relationship between parent and nurse and limitations must be acknowledged on both sides without fear of failure or inadequacy. The Practice Continuum (Figure 2.1) enables nurses in the practice areas to facilitate any aspect within the range according to individual need rather than a blanket approach that is not always achievable.

No involvement	Involvement	Participation	Partnership	Parent-led
Nurse-led	Nurse-led	Nurse-led	Equal status	Parent-led

Figure 2.1 Family-centred care: a Practice Continuum

The following three scenarios illustrate the use of the Practice Continuum according to differing individual family needs.

SCENARIO 2.1

John is a 3-year-old with bilateral chronic non-suppurative otitis media (also known as glue ear). Recent audiometry has revealed deficient hearing. The medical management of his problem involves an elective admission to the Day Care ward for bilateral myringotomies and insertion of grommets. John is an only child. It is his first hospital admission and he is going to be accompanied by his mother on the day of admission whilst his father goes to work.

The ward runs a pre-admission club one evening per week that families of children due for admission the following week are invited to for orientation purposes. During this visit the philosophy of family-centred care is explained to the families and brief video illustrations are used to highlight ways in which families may choose to be involved in their child's care on the day of admission. Families are encouraged to discuss any aspect of this that they feel requires clarification for their individual needs with the nursing staff present who will provide privacy if required. This serves to avoid expectation–experience mismatches between parents and nurses on the day of admission. An attractive backup leaflet (available in several languages appropriate to the local community) is given to parents before they leave and they are encouraged to telephone the ward with any further questions prior to admission.

Inevitably limited time is given to individual families at the pre-admission club and not all families are able or choose to attend, therefore the nurse admitting the child the following week may not be familiar to the family, although this would be ideal. So when considering the nurse and family relationship on the day of admission, they still meet as described by Hutchfield (1999) as relative strangers. Due to residual parental unfamiliarity with the environment and lack of specialist knowledge and skills in the area of safe pre and post-operative care, then the relationship between the nurse and parent is likely to be nurse-led. This may take the form of the nurse asking John's mother if she would like to bring him to the bathroom to get weighed pre-operatively, or suggesting that it is alright to lift John out of bed and cuddle him on her knee when he appears a little distressed post-operatively.

John's nursing needs are assessed on admission to the ward; this process may have been commenced at the pre-admission club. Operating in the belief that John's mother is what Hutchfield (1999) describes as the constant in John's life and the one who is intimately conversant with his needs, then the nurse draws on this maternal expertise when assessing his pre and post-operative nursing needs. His mother may be asked, for example, what particular words he uses to indicate his toilet needs or what she thinks John understands about what is going to happen to him today.

John's mother plays with him, sings nursery rhymes, looks at storybooks and helps him into his theatre clothes pre-operatively. She has previously indicated her wish to accompany John to the anaesthetic room. When he appears to be reluctant to get onto the trolley to take him to theatre, she automatically picks him up to reassure him and his nurse indicates that it's perfectly acceptable to carry him instead. John's mother continues to support him emotionally in the anaesthetic room as she follows his nurse's lead in talking softly to him and stroking his head in a soothing manner whilst the anaesthetist administers the anaesthetic.

Communication which is open and honest is essential to the relationship between the nurse and parent, which no matter how superficial it is initially, has a chance to develop and deepen over the period of hospitalization. Sometimes John's mother requests information, for example when walking back to the ward with his nurse she asks if John will cry when he 'wakes up' and if he is likely to be sick. More often than not, however, it is the nurse who sensitively takes the lead on carefully spaced information-giving as she prepares John's mother for the various stages of his pre and post-operative care. Later on, prior to John's discharge, information that has been discussed verbally such as how to avoid getting too much water in John's ears, is also supported with written advice.

Following John's return from theatre his mother retains her normal advocacy role by informing his nurse that he appears uncomfortable and acquiring appropriate pain relief for him. John's mother continues to support him emotionally post-operatively by cuddling him on her knee. She feels involved in his care as she continues her normal roles, for example giving him drinks and toast when his nurse has indicated that it is safe to do so. The nurse continues to give nursing care such as monitoring John's vital signs post-operatively.

The level of family-centred care achieved on the Practice Continuum in this instance was that of parental involvement, which was nurse-led (Figure 2.2). In the 5 or 6 hours prior to discharge the necessity for specific nursing input in certain areas only happened once e.g. the application of local anaesthetic cream prior to venous cannulation and the monitoring of pulse rate only continued for several hours post operatively. The requirement for these was relatively short-lived and it could therefore be argued that there was little to be gained in encouraging John's mother to participate further with them. She had made a valid contribution towards minimising the discontinuity described by Savage (2000) by being involved at this point on the Practice Continuum.

This is not a strict definitive example because John's mother could have chosen to be involved in more of his care, for example in the application of

No involvement	Involvement	Participation	Partnership	Parent-led
Nurse-led	Nurse-led	Nurse-led	Equal status	Parent-led

Figure 2.2   Diagram illustrating John's mother's position on the Practice Continuum

the local anaesthetic cream, or her personal strengths may not have included her confidence in feeling able to support John in the anaesthetic room. Although largely functional in nature at this stage, holistic elements are, however, apparent because the nurse respects and values whatever John's mother chooses to offer the situation, and the beginnings of a collaborative relationship (albeit brief) start to emerge.

SCENARIO 2.2

David is a 7-year-old boy with a 3-day history of periorbital oedema on waking. Initially his parents are not too concerned about this because the oedema disappears later in the day. However, when David returns home from school today saying that his socks hurt his legs and that his trousers are tight, a closer inspection by his mother reveals that David has a swollen abdomen and ankles. Following a urine test that reveals proteinurea at his general practitioner's surgery, David is referred to the children's medical ward for further investigations of what is provisionally thought to be nephrotic syndrome.

David and his mother are greeted by his nurse. She quickly perceives their anxieties about not yet having had chance to inform David's father of his son's admission. David's 13-year-old brother James is playing football in a school match with their father there as a keen supporter. Recognizing that this anxiety could hinder good communication and that David is not too ill, his nurse first directs them to the ward telephone kiosk. She suggests that if they are leaving an answerphone message for David's father to come to the ward, to ask him to bring David's clothing and toilet requisites with him and some for David's mother too, should she want to stay. The nurse takes the directional lead at this point due to David and his mother's unfamiliarity with the ward environment, routines and philosophy of family-centred care. Following this they are much more relaxed and open to assist in the admission procedure for David.

During David's admission the ward's philosophy of family-centred care is explained by his nurse, who also gives some brightly-coloured ward information leaflets for future reference to his family. She asks open questions firstly of David and then of his mother in order to gather data for the assessment of David's nursing needs. Already David and his mother start to feel that they are being listened to and that their contribution (although as yet

No involvement	Involvement	Participation	Partnership	Parent-led
Nurse-led	Nurse-led	Nurse-led	Equal status	Parent-led

Figure 2.3   Diagram 1 illustrating David's family's current position on the Practice Continuum

only verbal) is being valued (Figure 2.3). After discussion with David's father when he arrives, David's mother decides to stay in order to give her son emotional support and to continue some of her normal parenting role. David's father attempts to do the same for James at home so that the discontinuity of care described by Savage (2000) is felt less acutely by both children.

David's oedema and weight continues to increase generally over the next few days and the diagnosis of nephrotic syndrome is confirmed for which he is prescribed oral prednisolone. His nurse has a major role in information-giving at this point and answers questions openly and honestly about the medical condition and its implications for David. He settles quickly on the ward and his nurse decides to negotiate involving him and his mother in more of the hitherto nursing aspects of care. Both of them become quite good at working out how best to ration out David's restricted fluid intake across the span of his waking hours and recording the same on his fluid balance chart. They are also keen to take responsibility for measuring and charting urine output. The nurse teaches David's mother how to test the urine for blood and protein because she is likely to be asked to continue doing this when David is discharged. By the end of the first week of David's hospitalization although there is no improvement in his nephrotic syndrome, there is a good rapport established between nurse, David and family, which is collaborative in nature. The nature of care at this stage remains largely nurse-led but it has moved along the Practice Continuum from the stage of parental involvement to that of parental participation (Figure 2.4). The nurse is, however, still responsible for ensuring all care is given.

David spends a second week in hospital and although his condition does not deteriorate, little improvement is seen with the nephrotic syndrome. This week is further complicated by David's mother becoming ill herself with influenza and having to go home to look after her own health needs. Fortunately, David is not too upset by this and he is quite well-occupied in the daytime by the school teacher, nursery nurse and his own nurse. His brother visits on the way home from school and they watch football videos together. When David's father visits in the evenings he mainly chats and plays board games with David, but he is reluctant to get involved in urine testing and the recording thereof (Figure 2.5). David's nurse continues to give and be responsible for nursing care, for example daily weight and blood-pressure measurements as well as assisting with his hygiene care

No involvement	Involvement	Participation	Partnership	Parent-led
Nurse-led	Nurse-led	Nurse-led	Equal status	Parent-led

Figure 2.4 Diagram 2 illustrating David's family's current position on the Practice Continuum

(especially to oedematous skin folds), restricted fluid intake, low salt, high protein and carbohydrate diet, maintenance of fluid balance, urine testing and drug administration. She also ensures that David is able to chat with his mother by telephone each day.

No involvement	Involvement	Participation	Partnership	Parent-led
Nurse-led	Nurse-led	Nurse-led	Equal status	Parent-led

Figure 2.5 Diagram 3 illustrating David's family's current position on the Practice Continuum

Fortunately, good progress with the nephrotic syndrome starts to be seen in the following week, which is marked by a gradual diuresis and slow reduction in oedema. David's mother who has largely recovered from her influenza visits for most of the day, but goes home with his father in the evening. She quickly resumes her parental role and participates in nursing care as previously but also takes responsibility for David's diet and medication, following appropriate teaching from the dietician and his nurse. By the time David is discharged at the end of the third week, his mother feels empowered to meet David's continued nursing needs at home (Figure 2.6). With a now more equal relationship between nurse and parent, the nurse's role changes during the last few days of David's stay to that of supporter, advisor and facilitator. However, in this role the nurse is particularly careful not to focus just on David but shows her concern for all of the family. She recognizes that David's mother is still tired following her influenza and negotiates with her to take appropriate breaks off the ward. She is also careful to check that James is not feeling left out because she has noted that he has only visited once this week. Football matches and homework do, however, seem to be the main reason for this. David's father says it will simply be so much easier all round when everyone is back under the same roof again.

The level of family-centred care achieved on the Practice Continuum in this instance was that of parental involvement initially, progressing to parent

No involvement	Involvement	Participation	Partnership	Parent-led
Nurse-led	Nurse-led	Nurse-led	Equal status	Parent-led

Figure 2.6   Diagram 4 illustrating David's family's current position on the Practice Continuum

participation both of which were nurse-led during the first week. It did not matter that it moved back to parent involvement during the second week because it was more important at that stage for David's father to concentrate on continued emotional support of his son rather than feeling pressurized to acquire new skills (for example the urine testing that his wife had previously done). The contribution made by David's father and brother during this time was very worthwhile. As maternal confidence grew and more participatory skills were acquired during the last week, the power base was starting to shift from being nurse-led to being parent-led, and a more equal status between the two was starting to emerge suggesting a progression along the Practice Continuum towards a more parent-led partnership.

Again this is not a definitive example but it demonstrates that families can move in either direction on the Practice Continuum in accordance with their unique needs week by week, day by day or hour by hour if necessary.

SCENARIO 2.3

Susi is a 13-year-old who came from Hong Kong with her mother and 10-year-old brother Thomas to join relatives in England following the death of her Chinese father two years ago. The family speaks good English, but Thomas has had some bullying at school related to his ethnic origin which has made settling in a foreign country difficult. Susi's mother works regular hours for a city finance company, which largely fits in with the children's school hours.

Following a report from the school teacher that Susi has started to experience problems in seeing the classroom chalkboard clearly and, more recently, has needed to leave class to go to the toilet quite frequently, Susi's mother takes her to their general practitioner and also informs him of Susi's lethargy and thirstiness. A blood test revealing hyperglycaemia and a urine test showing glycosuria and ketones result in Susi being admitted to the hospital's adolescent unit with a diagnosis of diabetes mellitus.

Susi's admission is nurse-led (Figure 2.7) because her and her family are unfamiliar with the ward environment and what may be required of them. The philosophy of family-centred care is explained to them and Susi's

No involvement	Involvement	Participation	Partnership	Parent-led
Nurse-led	Nurse-led	Nurse-led	Equal status	Parent-led

Figure 2.7 Diagram 1 illustrating Susi's family's current position on the Practice Continuum

nurse collects data initially from Susi and then her mother in order to discuss Susi's current nursing needs with them and involve them in planning her care for the next few days. They have many questions about how diabetes will affect Susi's future lifestyle, which her nurse answers openly and honestly. She also gives them written information to reinforce what they have been discussing. Although Susi and her mother are initially devoid of knowledge and skills in the treatment of diabetes, which can make them feel powerless, they do however start to feel respected and involved through the process of consultation. On the evening of admission Susi's nursing needs of subcutaneous insulin injections, adequate carbohydrate and fluid intake, blood glucose monitoring and urinalysis are all performed by her nurse. Thomas has been very quiet since Susi's admission and her mother wishes to take him home. Their mother is acutely aware of her divided loyalties to the differing needs of her two children right now but when she sees the normally independent Susi involved in computer games with another patient, then the decision is made to go home with Thomas and return the following day.

The next morning Susi is visited by Jane the children's diabetes nurse specialist who will be advising on Susi's care in hospital and in the community when she is discharged home. It's now the weekend and when Susi's mother and brother arrive before lunch, they are surprised to learn that under the guidance of Jane, Susi has been taught to give her own insulin injection that morning. Throughout the weekend, Susi's nurse and Jane continue to establish a good rapport with Susi and her family. Following the on-call dieticians visit, they work collaboratively to gain an understanding of how to balance the required amount of insulin with the appropriate amount of dietary carbohydrate and exercise. The nurses take the lead in a step-by-step approach to gradually negotiate with Susi and her family increased participation in her care (Figure 2.8). This also takes the form of teaching them urinalysis and blood-glucose monitoring including how to act on the results. Once the signs, symptoms and treatment principles of hypoglycaemia and hyperglycaemia have been grasped at a rudimentary level, Susi's nurse explores the possibility of discharge with her and her mother. They agree that sufficient knowledge, skills and confidence are in place for this to happen on the Sunday evening. Also they feel reassured that Jane will visit them at home the next day prior to school to continue her supportive role and advise further, should that be necessary. Knowing that Jane or the ward may be telephoned for help at any time, Susi and her family are

No involvement	Involvement	Participation	Partnership	Parent-led
Nurse-led	Nurse-led	Nurse-led	Equal status	Parent-led

Figure 2.8 Diagram 2 illustrating Susi's family's current position on the Practice Continuum

excited to be going home and even Thomas eagerly helps to pack and carry some of Susi's belongings.

Susi settles into the 'diabetic routine' quite quickly and throughout the next year a caring partnership is forged between herself, her family and Jane (Figure 2.9). Jane is consulted quite frequently at first, for example advice is sought on the first occasion when Susi develops a cough and cold. The resulting hyperglycaemia in this instance being treated with an increased insulin and fluid intake, together with monitoring her blood-glucose levels more frequently. Continued contact with Jane provides the ongoing teaching that empowers Susi and her mother to feel knowledgeable, skilful and confident in all aspects of Susi's diabetic management. Home visits by Jane are gradually replaced by mainly telephone contact, which is now instigated by Susi's family when required, as they take the initiating lead instead of Jane. This shifting of power and control to the family and the 'sharing of mutually agreed roles' (Valentine, 1998, p. 26) results in a respectful partnership where Susi and family are the experts in how her diabetes affects them and Jane retains her broad and specialist children's nursing expertise.

In her role of caring for the whole family in the months following Susi's discharge from hospital, Jane is able to provide a forum where Thomas's mother can voice her concerns about her son's increasingly withdrawn behaviour and reluctance to communicate on anything other than a superficial level. In conjunction with their general practitioner, Jane is able to instigate some therapeutic sessions for Thomas with the clinical psychologist. In this 'safe' forum, Thomas is able to develop some useful strategies for dealing with what turns out to be some residual bullying at school. He is also helped to work through his irrational fears that now Susi has diabetes she will die like his father did.

No involvement	Involvement	Participation	Partnership	Parent-led
Nurse-led	Nurse-led	Nurse-led	Equal status	Parent-led

Figure 2.9 Diagram 3 illustrating Susi's family's current position on the Practice Continuum

In the two years following Susi's diagnosis, she and her family have become active members of the local branch of the diabetic association. Due to their now extensive knowledge and confidence of 'living with diabetes' successfully, they are currently involved in pioneering a befriending service for families of newly-diagnosed diabetic children in order to be able to offer family support in conjunction with the nursing support offered by Jane.

It can now be suggested that Susi and her family are at the point on the Practice Continuum that can be described as parent-led family-centred care. (Figure 2.10) The family themselves are experts on what it is like to live with Susi's diabetes and how to respond to the differing health challenges that can be presented by it on a daily basis. They have a mutually respectful relationship with Jane whose professional expertise they still choose to use in a consultative capacity from time to time. The family is also demonstrating their confidence by leading new initiatives and being involved in policy-making at the local branch of the diabetic association.

No involvement	Involvement	Participation	Partnership	Parent-led
Nurse-led	Nurse-led	Nurse-led	Equal status	Parent-led

Figure 2.10 Diagram 4 illustrating Susi's family's current position on the Practice Continuum

Summary

The provision of a contemporary definition of family-centred care in this chapter underpins the Practice Continuum and encompasses all the key elements of the concept. An explanation of different theoretical frameworks seems to reflect the evolution of the concept; it demonstrates the lack of theoretical clarity that has persisted and the difficulties this leads to in attempting to implement the concept of family-centred care in practice.

The contribution our Practice Continuum makes to both the theoretical debate and the practice of family-centred care is that it provides more clarity and flexibility to truly meet the needs of families and children. This has the advantage of respecting the validity of the family position on the Practice Continuum at any given point in time, as shown in the scenarios used in this chapter.

References

Ahmann, E. (1994) 'Family Centred Care: Shifting Orientation', *Pediatric Nursing*, March–April, 20(2), pp. 173–6.

Ahmann, E. (1998) 'Examining Assumptions Underlying Nursing Practice with Children and Families', *Pediatric Nursing*, September–October, 23(5), pp. 467–9.

Baker, S. (1995) 'Family Centred Care: A Theory Practice Dilemma', *Paediatric Nursing*, July, 7(6), pp. 17–20.

Bruce, B. and Ritchie, J. (1997) 'Nurses' Practices and Perceptions of Family Centred Care', *Journal of Pediatric Nursing*, August, 12(4), pp. 214–22.

Cahill, J. (1996) 'Patient Participation: A Concept Analysis', *Journal of Advanced Nursing*, 24, pp. 561–71.

Callery, P. and Smith, L. (1991) 'A Study of Role Negotiation Between the Nurses and the Parents of Hospitalised Children', *Journal of Advanced Nursing*, 16, pp. 772–81.

Callery, P. (1997) 'Caring for Parents of Hospitalised Children: A Hidden Area of Nursing Work', *Journal of Advanced Nursing*, 26(5), pp. 992–8.

Casey, A. and Mobbs, S. (1988) 'Partnership in Practice', *Nursing Times*, November 2, 84(44), pp. 67–8.

Casey, A. (1988) 'A Partnership Model with Child and Family', *Senior Nurse*, 8(4), pp. 8–9.

Casey, A. (1995) 'Partnership Nursing: Influences on Involvement of Informal Carers', *Journal of Advanced Nursing*, 22, pp. 1058–62.

Coyne, I. (1995) 'Parental Participation in Care: A Critical Review of the Literature', *Journal of Advanced Nursing*, 21, pp. 716–22.

Coyne, I. (1996) 'Parent Participation: A Concept Analysis', *Journal of Advanced Nursing*, 23, pp. 733–40.

Darbyshire, P. (1993) 'Parents, Nurses and Paediatric Nursing: A Critical Review', *Journal of Advanced Nursing*, 18, pp. 1670–80.

Darbyshire, P. (1994) *Living with a Sick Child in Hospital: The Experiences of Parents and Nurses* (London: Chapman & Hall).

Dearmun, A. (1992) 'Perceptions of Parental Participation', *Paediatric Nursing*, September, 4(7), pp. 6–9.

Dunst, C. and Trivette, C. (1996) 'Empowerment, Effective Help Giving Practices and Family Centred Care', *Pediatric Nursing*, July–August, 22(4), pp. 334–7.

Evans, M. (1994) 'An Investigation into the Feasibility of Parental Participation in the Nursing Care of their Children', *Journal of Advanced Nursing*, 20, pp. 447–82.

Graves, C. and Hayes, V. (1996) 'Do Nurses and Parents of Children with Chronic Conditions Agree on Parental Needs?' *Journal of Pediatric Nursing*, 11(5), pp. 288–99.

Hutchfield, K. (1999) 'Family Centred Care: A Concept Analysis', *Journal of Advanced Nursing*, 29(5), pp. 1178–87.

Kawik, L. (1996) 'Nurses Attitudes and Perceptions of Parental Participation', *British Journal of Nursing*, 5(7), pp. 430–4.

Neill, S. (1996) 'Parent Participation 2: Findings and their Implications for Practice', *British Journal of Nursing*, 5(2), pp. 110–7.

Nethercott, S. (1993) 'Family Centred Care: A Concept Analysis', *Professional Nurse*, September, 794–7.

Sainsbury, C. P. Q., Gray, O. P., Cleary, J., Davies., M. M. and Rowlandson, P. H. (1986) 'Care by Parents of their Children in Hospital', *Archives of Disease in Childhood*, 61, pp. 612–5.

Savage, E. (2000) 'Family Nursing: Minimising Discontinuity for Hospitalised Children and their Families', *Paediatric Nursing*, March, 12(2), pp. 33–7.

Shelton, T. and Smith Stepanek, J. (1995) 'Excerpts from Family Centred Care for Children Needing Health and Developmental Services', *Pediatric Nursing*, July/August, 21(4), pp. 362–4.

Valentine, F. (1998) 'Empowerment: Family Centred Care', *Paediatric Nursing*, February, 10(1), pp. 24–7.

Wright, L. and Leahy, M. (1994) *Nurses and Families: A Guide to Family Assessment and Intervention*, 2nd edn, Philadelphia, F. A. Davis, cited in Savage, E. (2000) 'Family Nursing: Minimising Discontinuity for Hospitalised Children and their Families', *Paediatric Nursing*, March, 12(2), pp. 33–7.

Part II

FAMILY-CENTRED CARE: CHALLENGES AND ALTERNATIVE PERSPECTIVES FOR THE TWENTY-FIRST CENTURY

3

Implications and Challenges of Family-Centred Care

Maureen Bradshaw

Introduction

The aim of this chapter is to critically analyse the philosophy of family-centred care and its practice in contemporary children's nursing. The analysis will highlight issues involved in transferring the claimed advantages of such care into practice in the light of factors in the workplace that impinge upon the ability of children's nurses to implement the philosophy in reality. The chapter aims to acquaint the reader with a breadth of issues that may need to be appreciated and addressed before family-centred care theory can be converted into practical reality.

The family, care and caring

In Chapter 2 it has already been highlighted that when the all-embracing nature of the term family-centred care is used to describe a multifaceted concept, then to some extent this can lead to confusion surrounding its application in practice. Likewise, some of the individual words constituting the term 'family-centred care' may also be potentially confusing or problematic. The word family for instance (who is the object and focus of the care to be given), may not be defined in the same way by the caregiver and the recipients of that care. Each will have their own understanding and life experience of what family

47

means to them and the two may or may not be congruent. The previously conventional family comprising married father and mother plus one or more children is not necessarily the dominant social norm any more. Therefore if children's nurses are to focus their care on the family, then who exactly constitutes the family for a particular child needs to be assessed on an individual basis before assumptions are made (Campbell and Glasper, 1995). In their expectations of what 'family' may comprise, children's nurses' expectations may need to extend beyond conventional heterosexual parenting relationships as well as considering single-parent families and reconstituted families. In a multicultural society, Mares, Henley and Baxter (1985) also warn that the effectiveness of healthcare is reduced when an ethnocentric view of family life is taken. The danger here being that different cultural values, beliefs and practices to do with the client family may not be recognized by nurses or, even worse, they may be rejected.

Within the term 'family-centred care', the word 'care' may also prove problematic for some. The *Concise Oxford Dictionary* (1999) defines care in terms of providing what is necessary for someone's health, welfare and protection. It includes being interested in others and being concerned to look after and provide for their needs. Again, care-givers and care-receivers may have very different ideas of what constitutes care, the biggest influence on this possibly being how care has been modelled to them in their own life experience thus far. With reference to Maslow's (1970) hierarchy of needs, some may, for example, feel cared for if basic needs like those for food, water, warmth, shelter and being physically pain-free are met. Others, however, may only feel cared for if additional emotional and self-aspirational needs are satisfied. Children from families that are concerned, loving, supportive and appropriately protective may have had different experiences of care to others from chaotic and dysfunctional family backgrounds which may have required some 'care' to have been given by a variety of local-authority agencies. These differing notions and experiences of care can therefore amount to it being a less than straightforward thing to be aiming to deliver in a family-centred care context.

Another commonly held assumption that may interfere with the operation of family-centred care in practice is that every family is caring. Headlines in the mass media every week declare that this is not the case. At one end of the scale they report heroic attempts by some families to raise funds to secure potentially life and quality-enhancing treatments for ill children, however the same media also reports murder, child abuse and neglect by family members at the other end of the scale. In-between these two extremes, families vary enormously in the amount, level or quality of care that they are able or desire to offer each child. However, such families are nonetheless the usual primary care-givers in the community situation.

Care by parent vs family-centred care

There may also be a problem with the assumption that family-centred care is the same thing as care by parent. This may be true for many, and indeed the Children Act (Department of Health, 1989) believes that children are generally best looked after within a family with both parents playing a full part. However, under the provision of the same Act where the welfare of the child is paramount, it may be in the best interests of some children to be looked after by the local authority. Therefore local authority staff in a residential home may provide everyday 'family care' for some children, or alternatively foster parents are responsible for the provision. Legal guardians may give other children family care or it may predominantly feature grandparents, siblings and child-minders.

Nurses' knowledge and understanding of the concept

Numerous studies describe the problems encountered by children's nurses and families because of their potentially diverse understandings of what constitutes family-centred care. It has already been described in terms of parental involvement (Nethercott, 1993), parental participation (Neill, 1996) and partnerships between nurses and families (Casey, 1988), all or any of which may be perceived as family-centred care by either party. Add to this the differing nursing views as to whether it is a functional or holistic phenomenon (Hutchfield, 1999) and there is much scope for confusion. So how can this be addressed?

The challenge for student and qualified children's nurses is to continue to keep abreast of the breadth and depth of the evolving concept of family-centred care as research assists it to unfold in the twenty-first century. Ward nursing teams need to be afforded time to formally reflect on their family-centred care periodically (at least annually), and in the light of current research it may be necessary to debate afresh, agree and define the concept for their particular ward or unit. Debate and agreement are necessary if the concept is to be owned by all individuals and to really 'live' in practice. Bruce and Ritchie (1997) point out that simply espousing the philosophy does not ensure that it will be practised. When not being observed, nurses may therefore have a tendency not to practice elements of the concept that they personally have not 'bought into' or feel little ownership of.

Family-centred care is, however, likely to be defined somewhat differently between wards and units. This is because in reality there may, for example, only be opportunity for parental involvement during a five-hour stay on a day-care ward, hence the concept for this type of ward is likely to be defined in terms of parental involvement. However, a ward caring for chronically-ill children who sometimes have long or frequent admissions, may have opportunities to develop real working partnerships with children and families and partnerships may therefore be the focus of their definition of family-centred care. Both definitions will, however, be valid in the wider context of family-centred care. This also illustrates why it may be difficult to provide a common children's hospital or children's unit definition that all can usefully use. The illustration in Chapter 2 of the Practice Continuum, underpinned by our contemporary definition, would however be useful here to show how both definitions belong to the same overarching concept and have equal worth.

Diverse views on family-centred care and the implications for practice

Even if it is possible for all nurses on a ward to have a congruent understanding of family-centred care, there remains the problem that nurses and parents often have very diverse views on the meaning of the concept. This can result in poor understanding of each other's perspective and discrepant expectations of each other (Knafl *et al.*, 1988, cited in Bruce and Ritchie, 1997). Families therefore 'need to have a clear idea of the philosophy of the ward into which their child is admitted' (Campbell and Glasper, 1995, p. 28). This may mean that the philosophy, written clearly and simply in lay-person's language, is clearly displayed in communal areas of the ward in several languages appropriate to the hospital's catchment area. If the same information was used in the ward information leaflet, then this could be used in a preparatory fashion for families whose child was being admitted electively. It could also be used in a supportive manner for families whose child was admitted as an emergency. However, simply distributing the philosophy in writing is not enough. Nurses need to be conversant and confident with the philosophy themselves and committed to actively discussing and exploring its meaning for individual families on admission and subsequently.

Once the philosophy has been shared and some initial mutual understanding gained, the expectation of family-centred care is that the negotiation of care and roles will take place between nurses and carers. Much is written about the limited extent to which nurses really do negotiate, their limited skills in this area and influential factors (Kawik, 1996; Callery and Smith, 1991). Neill's (1996) study demonstrated that parents wished to participate in their children's care at a level of their own choosing. However assuming that all families are completely comfortable with making choices could occasionally lead to problems. Cognitive development, as the progression into adulthood is made, includes coming to terms with the fact that many of life's questions, issues and challenges can no longer be seen in absolute black or white terms and the shades of grey in between start to be appreciated (even if somewhat uncomfortably at first). There may not be totally right or absolutely wrong answers to some decisions and choices that nurses may wish to involve families in. Choice is about deciding on a course of action; it involves selecting out and deciding between alternatives. Making choices has consequences and adults are generally held responsible and accountable for the choices that they have made. This potential responsibility and accountability may be unwelcome in some families who are not accustomed to practising it and who would prefer the consequences of any decisions or actions taken as a result of choices to be someone else's responsibility (or fault as the case may be!). Other families who are normally confident in being accountable for their choices may temporarily feel less confident and out of their depth when feeling uncertain or threatened by the child's illness. The nurse therefore requires much skill and sensitivity when attempting to negotiate care and choices with families.

The idea of nurses negotiating care and involvement with families sounds good in theory but is often less than successful in practice. Nurses failing to recognize and respect parental expertise as care-givers is just one of the problems in this area. Also nurses are not always totally comfortable with sharing the care that they have traditionally given (Kawik, 1996). Student nurses in Baker's (1995) study, for example, wanted to practice care skills, especially technical ones themselves. They felt comfortable with parents doing 'mothering' jobs, but technical jobs and nursing tasks were seen to fit firmly in the nurses' domain. There was a fear here that if parents gained nursing knowledge then nurses would no longer be professionals and their traditional control over nursing work would be lost. Callery and Smith (1991) point out that the nurse on familiar territory, in control of information, with no special emotional ties to the child, is in a position to control the nurse–parent relationship. Should the nurse choose not to negotiate, then the parent is not in a strong position to take the initiative. Where there was a lack of communication, parents were unsure of what they were supposed to do and did not initiate care or spontaneously join in nursing procedures (Baker, 1995).

Why nurses want to be in control and barriers to relinquishing control to families (or at least sharing it) is worth exploring further. The ever-evolving philosophy of family-centred care is always a step (or several) ahead of commonly held beliefs, their resultant attitudes and the outworking thereof in practice. Nurses traditionally have ascribed to and functioned under a medical model of care where they have been educated to expect that they are the experts that oversee care. Accordingly, they have assumed responsibility for orchestrating care under the direction of physicians and the institution (Bruce and Ritchie, 1997). It could be argued that vestigial elements of this have been hard to shake off as nurses have moved from medical to nursing models of care.

Even the nursing process whilst focusing on patient needs, can still be operated in such a way as to leave the nurse firmly in control when it comes to determining how those needs will be met.

Children's nurses have also been required to make a further transition, this time into family-centred models of nursing care. The well-entrenched belief of nurse as expert is however a piece of unhelpful baggage that is not easily left behind as this transition is made. There has to be clarity, however, about what it is that the nurse is required to relinquish in order to practice family-centred care successfully. It is not nursing expertise that is to be left behind (we need as much of that as we can get), what has to be left behind is the belief that the nurse is the only expert. New beliefs have to be embraced by nurses at this point, namely that the family are also often experts on their child, however nurse and family may well be experts in meeting different aspects of the child's needs at their initial meeting. When these two experts pool their expertise there is much potential for them to become a powerful force in effectively meeting not only the needs of the child but also those of the whole family. This is a philosophical shift that requires fundamental development of personal beliefs and values on the part of children's nurses. If they do not really believe it, it will not come out of their mouths and fingertips in what they say and do in practice, and consequently control will not be shared with and relinquished to families. Nevertheless, when nurses are prepared to share and relinquish control and work collaboratively with families, Kawik (1996) suggests that it is possible for both parties to share the same assumptions and value each others contribution without fear or recrimination.

It is important to appreciate that being prepared to relinquish control to families does not mean saddling them with responsibility and accountability for aspects of care that they as yet have scant knowledge of or skills in. This is why the negotiation process (discussed in Chapter 6) is so important in unveiling initially and then subsequently what both families and nurses can offer the current situation. Nurses then have to be alert to the possibility that what the family *can* offer may not be the same thing as what they *choose* to offer right now, and that families may or may not wish to share the rationale for their choice with the nurse. Parental choice for no or minimal participation during a nursing shift may be due to many reasons, for example lack of confidence, exhaustion from caring for a sick child at home, or wishing to go to a party instead. Nurses, though, have to guard against putting their personal value judgements on to these choices of others if a valuing and respectful relationship with families is to be fostered. When inclusion in care to a desired level is the family choice, then role clarification and documentation thereof is imperative so that all concerned are clear and comfortable with who is doing what, when and whose responsibility it is. Ongoing evaluation of care and use of the Practice Continuum suggested in Chapter 2 should enable roles and levels of care participation to change by mutual assent, week by week, shift by shift or hour by hour as sick child and family needs dictate.

Nursing documentation

Nursing documentation itself can be problematic if its development has not kept pace with the evolving concept of family-centred care. In some cases it may be due to institutional requirements to use standardized documentation (often adult-orientated) not being challenged. For evaluation purposes, when reflecting on the efficacy of documentation for promoting family-centred care, ward staff may benefit from interviewing new staff and students to the ward during their first shift and asking such questions as: 'If your mentor was not able to help you today, what do these documents require of you and guide you to do?' 'Who do you think they require you to talk to?' 'Whose thoughts and concerns do they require you to record?' 'How do you know if you are required to do anything and for whom?' 'Will anyone else be doing anything and if so what?' 'What do the child and family think about care and progress so far, how do you know?' This is not an exhaustive list and staff can formulate their own test criteria with reference to current family-centred care literature. The point is that the documentation, whether written or computerized, needs to be developed in such a way as to make the elements of family-centred care philosophy overt and an obvious requirement. This should then be a useful prompt and guide for the staff and also families using it. It is worth looking at care-plan documentation by Casey and Mobbs (1988) for an early illustration of how documentation can facilitate the recording of care that has been negotiated with the family. Since then, Casey (1993) comments that regular reviews of the documentation have ensured that changes in practice, for example improved discharge planning, have been accommodated. With reference to computer-based systems for care planning, Kawik (1996) stresses the need for them to enable nurses to negotiate care with parents and clearly identify the extent of care that parents may wish to undertake. She also states that this may require nurses to redesign the nursing documentation in order to attain this goal.

Managing the change

It has been alluded to earlier in this chapter that in managing the change involved in using an evolving concept, then the bottom-up approach is important. That is, that in order to make the concept work in practice on their ward or unit, then the shopfloor workers (nurses on the ward) have to personally value the concept and desire to see it worked out in practice. Their degree of success may in part be directly proportional to the level of commitment of the weakest believer in the concept. There is a sense in which the concept lives or dies in practice at this level, but ward staff's firm belief in the concept and valiant efforts to see it worked out in practice can be partially thwarted by a lack of managerial and organizational support. Without this it is very difficult to pioneer the outworking of the concept in practice at ward level. 'The extent of an institutions commitment to family centred care affects the operationalization of such practices' (Bruce and Ritchie, 1997, p. 220). Therefore, there has to be a strong commitment and message, from the top down, that family-centred care is an expectation. This in itself has to be more than a mere mention on the hospital or unit's mission statement if simply paying lip service to the philosophy is to be avoided.

Management commitment to espoused philosophies and policies is usually judged by the shopfloor workers, in terms of the fruits that the commitment is actually seen to bear. So how can that managerial commitment be demonstrated in order that an appropriate leadership role may be taken in transferring the family-centred care philosophy into practice? Nurse managers who both know and believe in the philosophy of family-centred care must be prepared to fight for it by presenting an evidence-based rationale for its continuing development in strategic planning groups so that it is resourced appropriately both now and in the future. Declaring the philosophy on mission statements and standards documents will add weight to the managerial expectation that it is to be practised. However, if the standards and criteria against which the success of family-centred care is to be judged are created not just by managers but also by families and ward nurses, then there is real potential that such standards will be relevant and meaningful when audited. When auditing takes place it is imperative that it is done by the recipients of care as well as ward nurses. Therefore provision for doing this in several languages appropriate to the local community needs addressing if a truly representative view of the whole ward population is to be obtained. Bruce and Ritchie (1997) even suggest that if expectations of family-centred care were incorporated into annual nursing appraisals of performance, then this could assist nurses in the recognition of their accountability for such care. This suggestion has relevance not only for ward nurses but also their senior management.

Resourcing family-centred care appropriately is another way in which managers can demonstrate their commitment to it. The whole multitude of issues that this involves range from provision of appropriate accommodation and fair-priced food for resident families, to the provision of enough skilled children's nurses being granted the time to really put the theory into practice. Classroom discussions with student nurses and research by Bridgeman (1999) all highlight lack of time as a major inhibitory factor to the outworking of family-centred care in practice. Resourcing of staff also involves commitment to their continuing education on family-centred care through in-service training and releasing staff for relevant study days, conferences and courses.

Long-term vision is required by nursing and hospital managers regarding investing resources in family-centred care now in order to profit from this in the future. The short-term cost involved in resourcing the empowerment of nurses, who in turn can empower families through such care, is likely to pay long-term dividends in terms of increased future quality of family health and potentially reduced hospital expenditure as families take the lead in care in the future.

A multidisciplinary philosophy?

One of the difficulties encountered in implementing family-centred care from time to time is that it is not necessarily a multi-disciplinary philosophy. In areas where nurses have been diligent in implementing such a care philosophy, they sometimes find their efforts thwarted by other professional colleagues who do not value and operate within the same philosophical framework when visiting the ward, or when families visit other departments or hospitals. This can be quite confusing for families and can in some instances damage therapeutic progress and trust relationships that were being built. Interestingly enough, though, students often share anecdotal evidence of where the converse appears to be true sometimes. Here it is nursing colleagues who seem keen to restrict family involvement in care when other colleagues in the multidisciplinary team appear not to have a problem with it.

Creative but practical ideas are therefore required if family-centred care is to have value as a multidisciplinary philosophy in the future. One suggestion for assisting this to happen is the use of interdisciplinary teaching and learning, especially at pre-registration level. It is important that all disciplines have the opportunity not only to critically analyse and debate the merits of the concept for use within their own discipline, but also to explore the potential advantages to families and staff if this became a multidisciplinary philosophy. If nurses are committed to working in a truly multidisciplinary arena it may even be possible to enhance multidisciplinary aspects of care by being involved in interdisciplinary research studying mutuality and collaborative relationships between families, children's nurses and colleagues in the multidisciplinary team. Further work may need to be done to ensure that more flexible approaches to care can be utilized by all and that hospital children's nurses are not working in isolation as they strive to implement family-centred care. This is because if the implementation of the concept in real life is going to benefit families, then it needs to evolve in a form where it can transcend boundaries in order to facilitate a more seamless web of care. The boundaries to be addressed may be cultural, those between disciplines and those between hospital and community.

Nurse education

Another issue for the future is that of nurse education, as it too needs to continue developing in order to keep pace with the evolving concept of family-centred care. There is evidence from Baker (1995) and Bruce and Richie (1997) that nurses have a good understanding and knowledge-base about family-centred care as a theoretical concept, but evidence from the same studies found that nurses experienced difficulty in translating this theoretical knowledge into practice for a variety of reasons. Nurses reported in one study a lack of adequate education to help them understand and practice such care particularly with reference to 'negotiation and sharing information with families and parental involvement in decision making and care planning' (Bruce and Ritchie, 1997, p. 218). The response of nurse education to such studies must be represented in curriculum development. Skills training in negotiation, empowerment and teaching must not only be present in nursing curricula, but they must now have a much higher profile in order to equip children's nurses of the twenty-first century, for translating family-centred care, theory into living practice. The 'what comes where' aspect of future curriculum development may also require consideration if it is not only to enhance the valuing of family-centred care, but also the ability to practice it in the real world and thus narrow the current gap between theory and practice. Several studies and student feedback suggest that students (and newly-qualified nurses) are valued by qualified ward staff primarily for their ability to perform physical nursing tasks, for example patient observations and interpretation thereof, administering prescribed drugs safely, ability to use suction apparatus in an emergency, and so forth. When these have been demonstrated satisfactorily, a sense of acceptance and belonging within that particular ward culture is often achieved. At this point of confidence and competence it may then appear more culturally acceptable for students to become free to concentrate on the less tangible and measurable aspects of care, for example the philosophical approach of family-centred care. Future curriculum planners may therefore need to plan for the acquisition of skills like safe aseptic technique and medicine administration early in educational programmes, in order that the opportunity to learn the equally practical and important family-centred care skills like negotiation and empowerment comes at the point when students are most open and freest to explore and learn those skills. Thought may also need to be given to the accompanying teaching methods as an increase in the use of videoing and role-playing, for example, may be required to assist in the development of some of the interpersonal skills necessary to negotiate family-centred care successfully.

A combined educational and managerial issue presenting a challenge for the future of family-centred care within children's nursing is that of post-basic education. Some children's nurses experienced no or minimal family-centred care input in their own pre-registration curricula. Further post-basic education opportunities may therefore be required in order to enable such nurses to further explore the current breadth and depth of the concept and the skills required to successfully practice family-centred care. Kawick (1996), for example, suggests that in order for the concept to be incorporated into practice, nurses may need to further explore their own values and beliefs. She suggests that both in-service training and continuous education programmes could act as the catalyst for this process by using reflection and encompassing such areas as family dynamics, role clarification and negotiation skills. Unless these nurses can be empowered to fully internalize the concept and feel confident in practising it, then it will continue to be difficult for them to lead from the front and be successful role models for junior staff in the area of family-centred care. Qualified staff have much power in shaping what their particular ward culture will allow family-centred care to be. Coleman *et al.* (2000/2001) point out that when there is a gap between students' knowledge of what such care could be and the reality of what the ward cultural environment allows it to be, then this can lead to cognitive dissonance which creates stress for students that they can well do without. Coleman *et al.* suggest that it could be seen as immoral or unethical to expect students armed with family-centred care knowledge to resist and change occupational culture on their own in this area and that qualified staff responsibilities on this issue need to be taken seriously.

Summary

Children's nursing has not stood still over the last 50 years and the development of family-centred care theory in all stages of its evolution has already influenced many positive developments in children's nursing practice. However, we have not yet arrived at that destination where there is satisfaction that all aspects of a family-centred care philosophy are being implemented efficaciously in practice, and so the pioneering journey must continue. Children's nurses are therefore required to take ownership of their responsibility to wrestle with the unresolved issues discussed in this chapter, until the barriers to successful implementation of such care are broken down and it becomes a living reality.

The following critical review of parenting in society in Chapter 4 will continue to raise issues from our ever-changing society that require family-centred care to be equally dynamic in nature in order to keep pace.

References

Baker, S. (1995) 'Family Centred Care: A Theory Practice Dilemma', *Paediatric Nursing*, July, 7(6), pp. 17–20.

Bridgeman, J. (1999) 'How do Nurses Learn about Family Centred Care'? *Paediatric Nursing*, May, 11(4), pp. 26–9.

Bruce, B. and Ritchie, J. (1997) 'Nurses' Practices and Perceptions of Family Centred Care', *Journal of Pediatric Nursing*, August, 12(4), pp. 214–22.

Callery, P and Smith, L. (1991) 'A Study of Role Negotition between the Nurses and the Parents of Hospitalised Children', *Journal of Advanced Nursing*, 16, pp. 772 – 81.

Casey, A. (1988) 'A Partnership Model with Child and Family', *Senior Nurse*, 8(4), pp. 8–9.

Casey, A. and Mobbs, S. (1988) 'Partnership in Practice', *Nursing Times*, 84(44), pp. 67–8.

Casey, A. (1993) 'Development and Use of the Partnership Model of Nursing Care', in Glasper, E. A. and Tucker, A. (eds), *Advances in Child Health Nursing* (London: Scutari).

Campbell, S. and Glasper, E., A. (1995) *Whaley and Wong's Children's Nursing* (London: Mosby).

Coleman, V., Bradshaw, M., Cutts, S., Guest, C. and Twigg, J. (2000/2001) 'Family Centred Care: A step too far?' *Paediatric Nursing*, 12(10), pp. 6–7.

Concise Oxford Dictionary (1999) Oxford: Oxford University Press.

Department of Health, (1989) *The Children Act* (London: HMSO).

Hutchfield, K. (1999) 'Family Centred Care: A Concept Analysis', *Journal of Advanced Nursing*, 29(5), pp. 1178–87.

Kawik, L. (1996) 'Nurses Attitudes and Perceptions of Parental Participation', *British Journal of Nursing*, 5(7), pp. 430–4.

Mares, P., Henley, A. and Baxter, C. (1985) *Health Care in Multiracial Britain* (Cambridge: National Extension College/Health Education College).

Maslow, A. H. (1970) *Motivation and Personality* 2nd edn (New York: Harper & Row).

Neill, S. (1996) 'Parent Participation 2; Findings and their Implications for Practice', *British Journal of Nursing*, 5(2), pp. 110–17.

Nethercott, S. (1993) 'Family-Centred Care; A Concept Analysis', *Professional Nurse*, September, 794–7.

4

Parenting in Society: A Critical Review

Gary Mountain

Introduction

Assumptions are made that the family (and by family, often read parents) is recognized as the most important contextual influence in human growth and development. Models, frameworks and philosophies of family/child-centred care all emphasize that the development, operability and outcomes of an individual child's care programme or pathway are heavily reliant upon specific factors, such as family system elements and in particular the adequacy of parenting. Similarly the majority of what is found in the literature about parenting typifies an ideal-type portrayal of married heterosexual parents displaying the natural behaviours and skills required for the successful socialization and development of their child(ren). This chapter aims to offer a critical framework through which to understand the complex theme of parenting. The discussion adopts both cross-cultural and social constructive perspectives and sets the analysis within a postmodernist agenda, viewing parenting and childhood as synonymous social constructs that have evolved with socio-historical changes.

The chapter will get the reader to explore the diverse nature of parenting and begin to question the general assumptions often made that the parental attitudes, behaviours and styles inherent in models of parenting and family-centred care are fundamentally altruistic and facilitative. Finally the chapter will help the reader to apply the key theoretical principles and concepts to practice.

Parent(mother)hood

Politicians, professionals and scholars have too often easily assumed that parenting is a natural phenomenon which individuals voluntarily assume and undertake easily, and that the needs of parents and their offspring somehow harmoniously coalesce to facilitate optimum childrearing (Skolnick, 1978, pp. 275–6). Parenting is rarely shared equally, with the major burden falling to women, and motherhood has been a key theme of many feminist and social constructionist critiques, as seen for example in Phoenix (1991) and Saraga (1998). The label of mother, like so many other labels in society, is so well-established or taken for granted as to be viewed as natural. The social constructionist would add a cautionary note in that the application of such labels carries deeply embedded patterns of social expectations. For example, there are socio-cultural assumptions that all women are or want to be mothers. Secondly, it is automatically assumed that 'mothers' will display the appropriate behaviours, love their children unconditionally, be attentive to their idiosyncratic needs and ensure they thrive despite the many challenging contexts they can find themselves in. Although she will receive very little or no coherent support or preparation for motherhood, if she abandons her responsibilities or even detracts from societies norms then we are likely to label her as 'unnatural' and seek to ascertain causes for her failings (Saraga, 1998).

Such views can also undermine the enormity of the task that so many parents (or more accurately individuals who carry the label mother) face when trying to give their children the best possible start in life. The effects of motherhood can include considerable physical, intellectual and emotional 'stressors' for those concerned, and many women will also carry the dual burden of trying to combine motherhood with work. It is well-documented that the concept of motherhood, and the interrupted employment patterns and opportunities associated, is still a key basis for gender discrimination in the workplace today, which in turn is one of the key factors for wider gender inequality in society.

Parent (father)hood

Any analysis of parenting should not only restrict its focus to mothers, but also address fatherhood. Nonetheless, we seem to know much less about the realties and perspective of fatherhood than we do motherhood. The sceptics among us are likely to begin to ask, 'can men mother with the same quality as their female counterparts and if so why don't men mother?'

Evidence would suggest that men can be competent care-givers, however in many cases men do not chose this as their main role due to the personal commitment and costs this would entail. Studies such as those by Lamb (1987) and Parke (1981) have found that whilst our society acknowledges the significance of the male contribution to parenting, beyond the newborn period fathers generally still continue to spend less time than mothers in the everyday care and welfare of the child. Nevertheless there is some evidence to suggest that the absence of the father figure can have negative outcomes for the child, for example in the emotional and cognitive domains (see Wallerstein and Kelly, 1980).

Fitzgerald, Mann and Barratt (1999) remind us not to forget the impact that fathers have on their infants and young children. The authors suggest six themes that are not only descriptive of contemporary parenting from a male perspective, but also represent an agenda for guiding future research into this topic. They concur that we need to focus on direct assessment of father's parenting behaviour, rather than relying solely on maternal reports. Just as we tend to investigate the influences of mothering, we need to also focus on the effects of fathers' presence on early child development, rather than the effects of their absence. Similarly there is a need to conceptualize the family as more than a dyad regardless of whether a biological or social father is part of the family unit. We need to explore and take cognizance of individual differences among fathers, including within-culture and cross-cultural determinants of fathering and their impact on child outcomes. Finally, there is a need to focus on the fathers' participation in gender socialization as well as psychotherapeutic interventions involving families with infants and young children.

Diversity in parenting

It could be argued that often what is known to date about parenting and parent–child relationships generally has been derived from limited myopic constructions of family as well as culturally-restricted samples (McCollum, Ree and Chen, 2000). Families have changed, as has the nature of the relationships within them (Beck, 1992), and contrary to popular belief this is not a consequence of the erosion of the family, rather, as what Jenks (1996) terms, part of the set of emergent conditions that have come to be collectively known as late or postmodernity.

The key changes within family structures that we have witnessed include the wide variation in the timing, number and spacing of births with some families established at the upper limits of a woman's fertility and some men becoming fathers at such an age that they may not see their children reach adulthood. Marriage is not necessarily an early temporal goal anymore, and is also a repeatable experience as witnessed in significant rises in divorce, lone parenting, reconstructed families, dual-worker families as well as the recent rekindling of the popularity of adoption and fostering (*Social Trends*, 1997). Whilst reconstituted families and reconstructed families confer membership to a new family and carry certain advantages for children, there will be in many cases, a wide range of challenges for them to overcome caused by a variety of transitions, transformations, disputes and periods of conflict experienced by both parent(s) and child(ren). Accepting that preparation for parenting generally is less than optimal in the UK, then for those individuals seeking preparation for re-parenting the picture appears rather bleak.

There are obviously other forms of diversity within family structures created by social class divisions, illness, culture and religion, sexual orientation of partners and the many alternative lifestyles coexisting within late modernism that are difficult to count.

In labelling a diverse form of parenting there is a danger that discrimination and inequality can at best be explained away, and at worst become justified. Whilst acknowledging that behavioural problems as well as other social actions displayed by children and young people can have their origins in parenting attitudes and behaviours (SolisCamara and Romero, 1996), contemporary political rhetoric still has a tendency to locate the impetus for some of the main problems associated with family life solely at the personal level of the parent(s) involved. Diversity in parenting almost permits others to locate problems within families as separate from the enduring nostalgic notion of the nuclear family. The media very recently reported that the mother of a persistent truant had been ordered to attend lessons on how to become a better parent! The Parenting Order was served on the mother after her son aged 14 turned up for school on only 39 days out of the possible 256. She faced a fine of up to £2000, but as an alternative magistrates decided to make her one of the first people to be bound by a Parenting Order. The Order requires the child and mother both to attend counselling sessions with police, social services, education services and a probation officer (De Bruxelles, 2000).

The contentious issues with regards to gay parenting are still hotly debated, but what is obvious is that along with teenager and/or lone parenting, such ideologies are perceived as less desirable. However, it is imperative that we begin to acknowledge the various practices and pathways of parenting and try to support those who are attempting to raise their children in a caring context. We must also consider society's views on lone parenting versus dual parenting. The former can often be cited as 'burdens on the state' and responsible for producing children more prone to low educational attainment, delinquency, unemployment and crime (see Dennis and Erdos, 1993). Whilst popular ideology presents lone parenting as 'less desirable' than dual parenting, it is important to consider the wide number of reasons why one parent may be absent; for example, working away, separation, divorce, widowhood, imprisonment or failure to acknowledge parenthood. Added to this are instances where one parent may have tried to escape bringing up their children in abusive or destructive environments.

Parenting also carries financial implications and a significant degree of high-quality involvement by those concerned. It is often difficult for dual working parents to cope with both paid work and time with their children, and for many single parents it is a continual up-hill struggle against multiple disadvantages. Added to this, a significant number of single parents are teenage mothers whose incomes from paid work (if at all) tends to be very much lower than those of men. According to Bernardes (1997), the way in which prejudice against poorer sections of society and ethnic minorities is combined is seen most clearly in the context of black single motherhood. Single mothers account for approximately 14 per cent of births in the general population compared with 51 per cent in the African-Caribbean population. Bernardes goes on to recommend that policies are urgently needed that lessen the enormous pressure and disproportionate chances of unemployment, poverty and parenting for our black citizens (Bernardes, 1997).

Differences in what is termed the 'emotional tone' of the family can have profound effects on the child(ren). As various reports suggest, children in warm and loving families are more securely attached in the first two years of life, have higher self-esteem, are more empathic, more altruistic, more responsive to others, and have a higher measured intelligence quotient in preschool and secondary school (Schaffer, 1989). They are also less likely to show maladjusted behaviour in adolescence and more likely to be responsive to guidance.

Some of the most influential proposals about patterns or styles of parenting and their influence on child development has come about from Baumrind (1967) and, more recently, from Maccoby and Martin (1983). Baumrind analysed combinations of four aspects of the dimensions of family interactions, namely: (1) warmth or nurturance, (2) level of maturity of demands, (3) the clarity and consistency of rules, and (4) communication between parent and child. Baumrind identified three specific combinations of these characteristics that culminate in three alternative styles of parenting: the permissive style that is high in nurturance, but low in maturity demands, control and communication; the authoritarian style which is high in control and maturity demands, but low in nurturance and communication; and the authoritative style that is high in all four.

Each of the above parenting styles is said to be linked with particular positive and negative outcomes. For example children growing up with permissive parents are likely to be more aggressive, immature in their behaviour with peers and in school, and less likely to assume responsibility and independence.

A more recent study of parental roles, styles and relationships of mothers and fathers in the Turkish culture by Sumer and

Gungor (1999) suggests that as compared to those from authoritarian and neglectful families, children reared in authoritative and indulgent families were more likely to have secure attachment (and less likely to have insecure attachment), high levels of self-esteem and self-concept clarity, and low levels of trait anxiety. A number of authors have expanded on Baumrind's categories to identify additional types. Maccoby and Martin (1983), for example, describe the neglecting or uninvolved type. In these cases parents are frequently physically uncaring and emotionally unavailable (through mental illness or addiction for example) to meet the needs of their children and have a tendency to be over-critical and condemning of their children. It follows that the most consistently negative outcomes can be associated with this style of parenting. Other types have been noted including 'affectionate-mentoring' and 'attachment' parenting. In the former, parents communicate unconditional love and affection for the child, and this love also includes guidelines and instructions in behaviour. Such parents tend to be self-confident, relaxed and firm in their management. The parents gradually relinquish responsibility to the child to enable her or him to make decisions based on the foundation information the parents have been providing. The child in turn learns to apply general principles to various situations; they learn discipline and acquire the skills to evaluate novel situations where guidelines are apparent. The child raised by affectionate-mentoring parents is said to develop security, life skills and self-confidence.

Critics assert that the complex nature of parenting cannot be restricted to three or four main parental styles. Parents use an eclectic approach to child-rearing, rather than just one, and different styles may be adopted at different phases of the parent/child relationship. It is worth highlighting that much of the research in this area is correlational and therefore it is difficult to conclude with certainty that parental style causes particular types of children's behaviour and/or outcomes.

The need for cross-cultural perspectives

There is an ever-growing demand for cross-cultural studies of parenting if we are to fully comprehend the complexity of this theme and use our knowledge in meeting the needs of parents and their children from an ever-changing diverse population. Central to the concept of culture is the expectation that different people possess different ideas and behave in different ways with respect to child-rearing. A study by Bornstein *et al.* (1996) investigated the perspectives that mothers and their partners from three different cultures held about child-rearing as well as what they considered to be ideal child-rearing. The results showed consistent parent, country, as well as parent-by-country effects, interpretable in terms of overarching cultural beliefs. The study helps professionals understand why and how parents from different cultures behave the way they do towards children, and provides insight into the broader social context of child development.

The variability of parenting activities found across cultures is because parenting constructs appear related to specific beliefs and socialization factors present in specific cultures. The ways of knowing and ways of acting which constitute a culture are constructed at both a collective and a personal level. Child-rearing provides frames of reference for parents' actions that in turn establish boundaries and guidelines for variability. Parenting contributes to the collective culture because it is a form of tacit expertise that entails the construction and modification of future behaviour (McNaughton, 1996).

The reader may find Bornstein's edited volume, *Cultural Approaches to Parenting* a useful additional evidence-based reference source on this vast topic. Universal and culture-specific features of child-rearing practices and socialisation are addressed using an array of methodologies across diverse cultural contexts. The text is useful in broadening the understanding of parenting and provides valuable insight into multicultural families and their children (see Bornstein, 1992).

The costs of parenting

Frequently portrayed in the literature are confident and powerful parents socializing their children and enjoying the pleasurable tasks and satisfaction associated with parenting (Zinn and Eitzen, 1990, p. 305). However, such ideologies ignore the direct and indirect economic costs of parenting and undermine the complexity of the interaction between parent(s) and child. The high emotional and financial costs paid by individuals (and more accurately mothers) in parenting and related tasks has been repeatedly calculated. Parenting demands a commensurate level of steady income to meet the considerable, ongoing and direct economic costs to parents in clothing, heating, feeding and so forth. Many studies have also identified the high emotional costs paid by women due to the high and continuous levels of interaction needed in mothering and related tasks. To this should be added the psychological implications of rearing children caused by the usual everyday problems children present such as sleeplessness, temper tantrums and disputes with adolescents (Umberson, 1989). Evidence would also suggest that a variety of quality measures in respect of marital/partnership quality decline in the parenting years, with the potential for conflict between being a parent and being a partner. The problems appear to be compounded when applied to teenage parenting. For example, four out of ten teenage mothers are said to suffer from depression within a year of giving birth – almost double the rate for single women of the same age living at home. They are also twice as likely to perceive themselves as being in poor health compared with their childless counterparts and report a diverse range of stresses (Social Exclusion Unit, 2000).

Despite the known pressures of parenting the UK compares poorly with the rest of the European Union in terms of maternity and paternity leave, maternity benefits and the provision of systemic support for parents and families. The New Labour Party in their recent consultation document openly admits that the UK fails to prepare young people adequately for parenthood and set out a raft of pragmatic measures aimed at tackling this longstanding issue (Home Office, 1999). Similarly, whilst one could argue that at least the ideological typifications of family and heterosexual parenting are beginning to be challenged, we still witness parents being solely blamed when children either do not develop as expected or fail to mature into 'well-adjusted young people'. Whilst the government has prided itself in announcing that three-fifths of the 177 manifesto commitments of 1997 have been fulfilled, it is questionable whether these political measures are going to be adequate to address some of the deep-seated problems children and families continue to face. For example Murray

(2000) argues that the laws on maternity leave are forcing women to return to work too early, and while recognizing the move towards creating polices to support parents caring for children, she would like the movement to be much more imaginative and be tailored to meet individual needs. It is only recently that the need for any systemic support for parents has been acknowledged.

Policy design also needs to recognize the persistence of poverty among families, which has been deemed the 'scar on the soul of Britain' (Brown, 1999). So many children grow up in poverty; their life chances and opportunities are severely thwarted and many of the poor children become poor adults and pass on the cycle of poverty to their children. Whichever longitudinal poverty concept is used, conclusive evidence shows that children, especially very young children, have high poverty risks compared to other groups in the population. For example using panel data from the British Household Panel Survey, Hill and Jenkins (1999) found that some 14 per cent of children were poor *at least three times* during a six-year interval (1991–96). The current Prime Minister has promised plans to end child poverty within 20 years and improve child welfare generally. These measures include proposals to help parents into work and to make work pay more for those in employment already (in particular around the minimum wage). The government has also introduced measures such as the working-family tax credit, integrated child credit, the Sure Start deal programme and the New Deals for lone parents. What is notable about these is that they are designed to help individuals make the transition from benefits to work rather than alleviating poverty by increasing out-of-work benefits. Hill and Jenkins (1999) go on to warn, however, that policies aimed to reduce chronic poverty using means-tested benefits will be compromised if benefits are targeted using information about current incomes. The effectiveness of government strategies and programmes has also been called into question in the recently published report by the Family Policy Studies Centre (2000). Reviewing the government's anti-poverty strategies it warns that while measures taken to date will address some of the problems, child poverty in Britain remains high. They identify that almost 2.2 million children live in workless households and that children living within some of our ethnic families are by far the poorest groups in Britain. Like many of their academic colleagues, the Family Policy Studies Centre concur that the focus on means-testing as a solution to poverty and social exclusion is likely to compound rather than relieve the problem.

Adolescent motherhood

Today, the UK has the highest teenage conception rate in Western Europe and one of the highest in developed countries. There are nearly 90 000 teenage conceptions a year in England resulting in 56 000 live births. Around 7700 of these conceptions are to under-16s (Social Exclusion Unit, 2000) with around one in eight women in Britain having a child before the age of 20 (HEA, 1999a). Ninety per cent of teenage births are outside of marriage, more than four times the rate in 1971. A significant number of young women who have their first baby in their teens go on to have a second child before they are 20. This translates into the fact that around 87 000 children in England today have a teenage mother (Social Exclusion Unit, 2000). Teenage pregnancy is frequently a cause and a consequence of social exclusion, and the risk of teenage parenthood is greatest for young individuals who have grown up in poverty, those with poor educational attainment and those leaving care.

Given such statistics it is important that we acknowledge the emergence of new family care-giving pathways and practices – those of adolescent motherhood. However, adolescent motherhood challenges what Lawson and Rhode (1993) term the 'politics of pregnancy' whereby society generally struggles over the appropriate age and marital status in which childbearing is to be encouraged, with clear overt disapproval when underage women bear children. The problem is further compounded when such a woman chooses to remain single and/or is black. There is little wonder, then, that many teenage mothers struggle to be recognized as a parent to their children. As the Health Education Authority and others have recently highlighted, a significant number of adolescents get little of the right kind of support (help back into education, and/or employment, help with attaining parenting skills), struggle to combat financial problems, experience relationship problems with the fathers of their children, have poor housing and drug or alcohol problems (HEA, 1999b; Social Exclusion Unit, 2000).

Yet there is a considerable body of evidence to suggest that many teenage lone parents would like to return to education and gain employment and, where they do, this will have a positive long-term effect on their child's welfare. Similarly, where family members generally, and parents in particular, are attuned to an adolescent mother's needs and are sensitive to her inexperience, mothering can engender a sense of purpose, significance and identity on behalf of the adolescent. Where parents have not learned to be receptive to their adolescent daughter's changing sense of self and agency, conflict ensues which dampens the adolescent mother's growth and maturity and hence precludes her from becoming a mother. Consequently the adolescent mother will be deprived of the space needed to experience her own decisions, emotions or emancipation except in reaction to her parents and possibly to her partner's will and arbitrary power (SmithBattle, 1997:148).

De-parenting and maternal ambivalence

Two important related concepts are worth noting. The former is where one or other parent becomes less involved in the parenting of a child and is said to follow de-partnering. This can be highly contentious for female partners, as society will have strong views when this involves de-mothering, perceiving it as absurd and unnatural. In terms of the latter, Parker has used studies of maternal ambivalence as a means of challenging motherhood. Similar to Skolnick's (1978) earlier postulation, motherhood and maternal development are frequently presented as misleadingly isomorphic when, in fact, it can often be characterized as consisting of pain, conflict and confusion created by the coexistence of feelings of love and hate within the mother. Parker goes on to categorize maternal ambivalence as being either manageable or unmanageable, and concurs that the former may even be a positive precursor to creative insight for the mother concerned as she attempts to make sense of her own feelings and others' responses (including that of her child) (Parker, 1997).

Parent–professional partnerships: integrating theory and practice

It is now widely accepted that parental participation and partnership approaches are pivotal concepts in the health and social care of children (Department of Health, 1989; Casey, 1988; Sainsbury *et al.* 1986). Although parental participation has a tendency to be still perceived mainly in terms of the mother's role, this may no longer be entirely appropriate for current health and social care practice as, due to the societal changes addressed in this chapter, many others may act as prime care-givers.

Practitioners working with children and their families must therefore have a knowledge and understanding of parenting within the contexts of childhood, family and caring for children. When we come to study parenting we will bring our own personal experiences and perspectives that in turn will undoubtedly shape some of our constructs. The reader therefore needs to approach the topic with an open mind. Understanding parenting involves a number of distinct elements. There is the centrality of parenting within the child's development, how this becomes shaped and constructed over time, and how diverse parenting can be. Whilst this chapter has provided the fundamental underpinning theory, integrating theory and practice can further enhance the reader's knowledge and understanding.

A very simple example in relation to the notion of parenthood is to identify some of the skills, abilities and qualities you think are needed to be a parent and then ask mothers who you come across what they think every mother should know before embarking on becoming a parent. Comparing your answers with those of others including peers may exemplify the diverse and complex nature of the topic. Secondly, it should encourage you to question how individuals are prepared for and supported through parenting. Contrary to the experience in the UK, preparation for parenthood is a common feature in many industrial societies. Undertaking some small-scale exploratory work in your local practice area should allow you to determine what investment in parenting programmes is being made in your local area and where is the political drive to improve parenting. No doubt the results of your work will reveal that a number of attempts have been made to establish a plethora of formal and semi-formal types of group-based parenting initiatives. However, these can often be confusing, uncoordinated and piecemeal, and fail to meet the specific individual needs of parents. Contrary to government ideology, evidence would suggest that parents do not always identify the need for specific parenting programmes, rather they prefer easy access to relevant healthcare professionals with whom they have developed effective relationships and therefore feel confident in approaching for support and advice (Wilbourn *et al.*, 2000).

Interpreting variation in family structure and parenting offers clear guidelines for devising family-centred care, partnership approaches and child-focused interventions. Having explored the diverse nature of parenting, practitioners should appreciate the importance of approaching such frameworks of care delivery in a non-judgmental way. Understanding the relatively 'normal' diverse patterns of parenting and the factors that are inextricably linked should mean that communication and collaboration with parents is more open, appropriate and facilitative. Working in partnership with families is not always easy and involves helping, facilitating and enabling both the child and parents in making a key contribution to the care and management of their child's health and social care. In order to do this effectively, the healthcare practitioner has to apply his/her knowledge of parenting and the specific characteristics, dimensions and/or styles that make up the parent–child interaction. They must apply their powers of observation and analysis and engage with the child and his/her parents so that true partnership approaches can be facilitated in an appropriate, meaningful and culturally sensitive way.

A second element covered in this chapter has been the costs of parenting, both in personal and economic terms. The reader should by now at least appreciate the demands imposed on individuals who are attempting to foster their child's optimum development under what can be challenging contexts, and also understand why and under what circumstances families can break down, and the effects of this on the child. Given what we know about the difficult task of parenting then it should not be difficult to deduce how the crisis of childhood illness and hospitalization can come to affect parents and other family members. The following discussion briefly reviews the various stressors and reactions of parents of a child who is ill and/or hospitalized including the alteration in parental roles.

The context of illness

Caring for a child who has an illness, whether at home or in hospital, can present a number of challenges for those involved. The more routine aspects of caring for a child can become more complicated, time consuming and emotionally laden (Eiser, 1990). For example, the problems associated with meeting the nutritional needs of infants and children can be a relatively normal aspect of everyday parenting, but when they occur in the context of illness the significance that feeding difficulties can take on can be of unprecedented proportions and can result in conflict between parents, and parent and child (Skuse, 1994; Drotar and Strum, 1988). Parents when trying to adjust and cope with the disruption that inevitably follows hospitalization, residency and follow-up care requirements can experience further stressors. Since the mother tends to be the main care-giver (Knafl and Dixon, 1984), she will spend a relatively longer period of time in the hospital than any other family member. However, it must be remembered that not all mothers adopt and adapt their role easily. Some may be under such stress that they need respite from total participation in care-giving. Others may feel insecure in meeting even the most basic care responsibilities in specialized healthcare environments.

Various studies have demonstrated that parents are willing to participate in direct care and emotional support of their child (Cleary, 1992); however, factors which frequently hinder participation include the healthcare practitioner's lack of attention to parent's needs, non-negotiation in care, and lack of information (Coyne, 1995). Thus parents and the family as a whole must be viewed within their relative social, cultural and religious contexts. Individual assessment of each parent and/or family members' preferred degree and nature of involvement is crucial while preventing negative interpretations of a parent's reluctance or hesitation to participate from evolving. Similarly, parents need to be both prepared and supported for the roles they choose to adopt. As mothers and fathers will each perceive different aspects of the child's hospitalization as stressful (Graves and Ware, 1990) and have different expectations of parental participation (Knafl and Dixon, 1984), their support needs will vary and support mechanisms will need to be tailored appropriately. The demands imposed by caring for a sick child means that s/he becomes the central focus of attention with the risk that family life revolves solely around the child at the expense of other family members. Similarly, the burden of balancing the demands and responsibilities of care-giving can create new tensions or strains on the family and relationships within it. These stresses and strains can be further complicated by the financial and social consequences for caring for a sick child. Consider, for example, the effects of a parent who already experiences financial difficulties who is forced to give up employment to care for his/her child and/or faces the additional expenses incurred due to travelling, the purchase of special equipment, the provision of adaptations to the home or special diets (see Fielding, 1985; and Breslau *et al.*, 1982). The effect of the child's illness on the family therefore needs to be assessed and bespoke support and care packages implemented.

The concept of parent participation can be seen to have evolved to embrace working partnerships with not only parents but also relatives and, more importantly, children themselves. These partnerships should reflect important attributes such as equality, mutual respect and decision-making. Parental attitudes and behaviours have a direct relationship with the social environment and decision-making of children across a diverse range of contexts. In the health and social care setting parents who demonstrate certain styles (e.g. adaptive) of parenting are said to foster the child's responsibility for self-care. Conversely, a manipulative style can result in tension and inconsistency. Such issues are important to note in instances involving decision-making by children, informed consent to care and treatments, as well as the integration of self-care.

Summary

This chapter has attempted both to convey and question the notion of parenting in current modern society. The brevity of this account is acknowledged; this complex topic merits further analysis in its own right. However, hopefully the discussion has illustrated how the personal and idiosyncratic worlds of parenting are not necessarily shared with those of the detached observer. Despite the plethora of competing critical debates on the subject, parenting continues to be understood and portrayed as being a naturally occurring and distinct feature for the majority of the adult (predominantly female) population in all societies. In addition there is an appeal to the idea that there is a natural way to parent, while at the same time the complex nature of parental roles and responsibilities are oversimplified. However, what should have become apparent from the preceding discussion are the key themes of diversity and variety.

Most recently politicians have begun to take cognizance of the diverse and complex nature of parenting and have noted some of the problems and issues that contemporary families face. Many of these centre on lone, working and marginalized families. This chapter has also highlighted additional compounding factors such as when a child becomes sick and or is hospitalized.

Key messages for those in the health and social care fields include the need to approach the study of parenting critically but non-judgementally. Ongoing debate as well as radical and novel approaches to the complex phenomenon of parenting are still needed so that we can offer effective, timely support and guidance for individuals. Accordingly, we need to apply and integrate the concepts and theoretical principles learned to the real world of practice. Many factors, some of which have been explored here, can create challenges and adjustment problems to the already demanding parenting role. The healthcare practitioner needs to take account of the impact these, particularly the impact if illness, can have on parents and families. Helping strategies need to be planned and incorporated within frameworks of care, which meet the diverse and complex challenges parents will inevitably face throughout various health–illness trajectories. Similarly, there is a need to recognize and anticipate how the demands and responsibilities of caring for a sick child can create an uneasy synthesis with everyday family life, and thus new tensions or strains for the family and relationships within it.

References

Baumrind, D. (1976) 'Child Care Practices Anteceding Three Patterns of Preschool Behavior', in E. M. Hetherington and R. D Parke (eds), *Child Psychology: A Contemporary Viewpoint*, 4th edn (New York: McGraw-Hill).

Beck, U. (1992) *Risk Society: Towards a New Modernity* (London: Sage).

Bernardes, J. (1997) *Family Studies: An Introduction* (London: Routledge & Kegan Paul).

Bornstein, M. H. (1992) *Cultural Approaches to Parenting* (Hove: Lawrence Erlbaum Associates).

Bornstein, M. H., Tamis-LeMonda, C. S., Pascual, L., Haynes, O. M., Painter, K. M., Galperin, C. Z. and Pecheux, M. G. (1996) 'Ideas about parenting in Argentina, France and the United States', *International Journal of Behavioural Development*, 19(2), pp. 347–67.

Breslau, N., Salkever, D. and Staruch, K. (1982) 'Woman's Labour Force Activity and Responsibility for Disabled Dependants', *Journal of Health and Social Behaviour*, 67, pp. 344–53.

Brown, G. (1999) cited by S. Jenkins in 'Persistent Pest', *The Guardian*, 8 March 2000.

Casey, A. (1988) 'A Partnership with Children and Family', *Senior Nurse* 8(4), pp. 67–8.

Cleary, J. (1992) *Caring for Children in Hospital: Parents and Nurses in Partnership* (London: Scutari Press).

Coyne, I. T. (1995) 'Partnership in Care: Parents' Views of Participation in their Hospitalised Child's Care', *Journal of Clinical Nursing*, 4(2), pp. 71–9.

De Bruxelles, S. (2000) 'Parenting Lessons for Mother of Eruants', *The Times*, 13 March, no. 66878.

Denis, N. and Erdos, G. (1993) *Families without Fatherhood* (London: Institute of Economic Affairs Health & Welfare Unit).

Department of Health (1989) *Children Act* (London: HMSO).

Drotar, D. and Strum, L. (1988) 'Parent–Practitioner Communication in the Management of Non-Organic Failure to Thrive', *Family Systems Medicine*, 6(3), pp. 304–16.

Eiser, C. (1990) *Chronic Childhood Disease: An Introduction to Psychological Theory and Research* (Cambridge: Cambridge University Press).

Family Policy Studies Centre (2000) *Family Poverty and Social Exclusion (Family Briefing Paper 15)*, Family Policy Studies Centre, London.

Fielding, D. (1985) 'Chronic Illness in Children', in F. Watts (ed.), *New Perspectives in Clinical Psychology*, Vol. 1 (Leicester: British Psychological Society Books).

Fitzgerald, H. E., Mann, T. and Barratt, M. (1999) 'Fathers and Infants', *Infant Mental Health Journal*, 20(3), pp. 213–21.

Graves, J. E. and Ware, M. E. (1990) 'Parent's and Health Professional's Perceptions Concerning Parental Stress During a Child's Hospitalisation', *Child Health Care*, 19(10), pp. 37–42.

80 Parenting in Society: A Critical Review

Health Education Authority (1999a) *Summary Bulletin: Reducing the Rate of Teenage Conceptions. An International Review of the Evidence: Data from Europe* (London: HEA).

Health Education Authority (1999b) *Summary Bulletin: Reducing the Rate of Teenage Conceptions. Young People's Experiences of Relationships, Sex and Early Parenthood: Qualitative Research* (London: HEA).

Hill. M. S. and Jenkins, S. P. (1999) *Poverty Among British Children: Chronic or Transitory?* Downloadable from Institute for Social and Economic Research website:www.iser.essex.ac.uk/pubs/worpaps/wp99-23.htm

Home Office (1999) *Supporting Families: A Consultation Document* (London).

Jenks, C. (1996) *Childhood* (London: Routledge & Kegan Paul).

Knafl, K. A. and Dixon, D. (1984) 'The Participation of Fathers in their Children's Hospitalization', *Issues in Comprehensive Pediatric Nursing* 7(4–5), pp. 269–81.

Lamb, M. E. (1987) *The Father's Role: Cross-cultural Perspectives* (Hillsdale, NJ: Erlbaum).

Lawson, A and Rhode, D. L. (1993) *The Politics of Pregnancy: Adolescent Sexuality and Public Policy* (New Haven: Yale University Press).

Maccoby, E. E. and Martin, J. A. (1983) 'Socialization in the Context of the Family: Parent–Child Interaction', in Hetherington E. M. (ed.), *Handbook of Child Psychology* (New York: Wiley).

McCollum, J. A., Ree, Y. and Chen, Y. J. (2000) 'Interpreting Parent–Infant Interactions: Cross Cultural Lessons', *Infants and Young Children*, 12(4), pp. 22–3.

McNaughton, S. (1996) 'Ways of Parenting and Cultural Identity', *Culture and Psychology*, 2(2), pp. 173–201.

Murray, L. (2000) *The Social Baby*, (London: The Children's Project).

Parke, R. D. (1981) *Fathering* (London: Fontana).

Parker, (1997) 'The Production and Purpose of Maternal Ambivalence', in W. Holloway and B. Featherstone (eds), *Mothering and Ambivalence* (London: Routledge & Kegan Paul).

Phoenix, A. (1991) *Motherhood: Meanings, Practices and Ideologies* (London, Sage).

Sainsbury C. P. Q., Gray O. P., Cleary J., Davies M. and Rolandson P. H. (1986) 'Care by Parents of their Children in Hospital', *Archives of Disease in Childhood* 61, pp. 612–5.

Saraga, E. (1998) *Embodying the Social: Constructions of Difference* (London: Routledge & Kegan Paul in association with the Open University).

Schaffer, H. R. (1989) 'Early Social Development', in M. Woodhead, R. Carr and P. Light (eds), *Becoming a Person* (Milton Keynes: Open University Press) pp. 5–29.

Skolnick, A. (1978) *The Intimate Environment: Exploring Marriage and the Family* (Boston: Little, Brown).

Skuse, D. (1994) 'Feeding and Sleep Disorder', in M. Rutter, E. Taylor and L. Hervsov (eds) (1997), *Child and Adolescent Psychiatry: Modern Approaches* (Oxford: Blackwell).

SmithBattle, L. (1997) 'Change and Continuity in Family Care Giving Practices with Young Mothers and their Children Image', *Journal of Nursing Scholarship,* 29(2), Second Quarter: pp. 145–9.

Social Exclusion Unit (2000) *A Report of Policy Action Team 12: Young People* (London: Stationery Office).

Social Trends, Central Statistical Office (1997) *Social Trends 1870–1997* (London: HMSO).

SolisCamara, P. and Romero, M. D. (1996) *Coherence of Parenting Atitudes Between Parents and their Children* Salud Mental 19(1), pp. 21–6, Institute of Mex Psiquiatria, Mexico City.

Sumer, N. and Gungor, D. (1999) 'The Impact of Perceived Parenting Styles on Attachment Styles, Self Evaluation and Close Relationships' *Turk Psikoloji Dergisi,* 14(44), pp. 35–62, Turkish Psychologists Association, Ankara.

Umberson, D. (1989) 'Parenting and Well-being: the Importance of context', *Journal of Family Issues,* 10(4), pp. 427–39.

Wallerstein, J. S. and Kelly, J. B. (1980) *Surviving the Breakup* (New York: Basic Books).

Wilbourn, V., Mountain, G., Smith, L., Wood, B., Green, H. and Manby, M. (2000) *Parenting in the Millennium: A Summary Report of an Exploratory Study into Parent and Health Visitor Perceptions of Parenting Programmes* (University of Huddersfield).

Zinn, M. B. and Eitzen, D. S. (1990) *Diversity in Families,* 2nd edn (New York: Harper & Row).

Part III

A TOOLKIT FOR PRACTICE: SKILLS AND GUIDELINES TO FACILITATE FAMILY-CENTRED CARE

5

Empowerment: Rhetoric, Reality and Skills

Valerie Coleman

Introduction

An attribute of the evolving concept of family-centred care in the twenty-first century is empowerment; there is an expectation that the use of a family-centred approach to care results in an outcome of empowerment for families. The Practice Continuum proposed in this book provides a theoretical framework within which families may be empowered at different levels. However, as demonstrated in Chapter 3, it is not easy for practitioners to translate the theory of family-centred care into practice, and as a consequence of this empowerment may not always be a reality for children and their families.

This is concerning because empowerment has been identified as a central tenet of health promotion (WHO, 1984, 1986, 1998). Downie, Fyfe and Tannahill (1990) suggested that people without power lack the autonomy and ability to make choices about their own lives and this does not promote health. It is believed that as an outcome of an empowerment process, individuals are able to take control of their lives and this results in the promotion of health.

Contemporary health policy (DoH, 1999) and nursing policy (ENB, 2000) all suggest that families should be empowered to take control over their own lives. The profile of childhood illness is changing and an increasing number of children are surviving with chronic conditions, and other children with acute illnesses are often admitted as day cases or are discharged home earlier than in past years. Therefore, nurses need to be empowering families to make health decisions and to give healthcare through partnership-working both in hospital and the community (ENB, 2000). Nurses also should be empowering the children themselves, especially those with chronic conditions, because the outcome of a successful empowering process in childhood would be an empowered adult (Hegar and Hunzeker, 1988). It is suggested by Igoe (1993) that self-sufficiency should be encouraged as part of the developmental process in childhood, as opposed to fostering passivity. This seems particularly pertinent in the twenty-first century when many children have to make the transition between child and adult health services and some of them seem to be experiencing difficulties with this move (CCHS, 1998).

'The concept of empowerment is both complex and slippery' (Tones, 1997, p. 40); empowerment is an ambiguous concept that lacks clarity and it has become an overused vague term in both health promotion and nursing practice. This may explain why the empowerment of families is not always a reality. The intention of this chapter is to clarify the meaning of the concept and then to explore empowerment both as a process and an outcome. A rationale will then be offered as to why empowerment rhetoric is not always translated into reality, prior to explaining how to empower families. There will be a focus on the skills of relationship-building with families, facilitation of participatory experiences and information-giving (and teaching). A scenario will be used to demonstrate how nurses can facilitate an empowering process.

Defining the concept of empowerment

Empowerment is a very complex and multidimensional concept, which is difficult to succinctly define. It seems to be 'a process of helping people to assert control over factors that affect their lives' (Gibson, 1991, p. 359):

> In simple terms, the concept of empowerment would appear to be the process of enabling or imparting power transfer from one individual or group to another. It includes the elements of

power, authority, choice and permission ... it is the result or product of the process of empowering. (Rodwell, 1996, p. 306)

Rissel (1994) argues that to some extent the meaning of empowerment may differ depending on the context and time in history. In the context of family-centred care, empowerment in the early evolution of the concept could have meant families asserting control over being able to visit their child in hospital, whenever they wanted to. Now in the twenty-first century it could mean families actually taking the lead in the management of their child's care. Defining empowerment becomes further complicated because it can occur at different levels on a continuum from individual empowerment through to community empowerment, and then on to political action (Robertson and Minkler, 1994). For most families self-empowerment at an individual level is the most likely outcome, but some families with sick children may achieve community empowerment through their membership of support groups like the Cystic Fibrosis Society and the Diabetes Association. Some of these families may proceed to take political action to gain adequate resources and care for their children.

Robertson and Minkler (1994) explain that there is a reciprocal relationship between the different levels of empowerment, which means that an empowered community facilitates the development of self-empowerment in its members. This suggests that for families to become empowered within the health service, both in hospital and the community, nurses themselves need to be empowered.

So what does empowerment mean? The rhetoric discussed here seems to suggest that it is: 'A reciprocal social process in which individuals and / or communities are helped to participate with competence, to take control over the factors that affect their lives' (Coleman, 1998, p. 32). Others have highlighted competency development as a prerequisite for empowerment, notably Rappaport (1985) who suggests that competencies are already present in most people and, given the appropriate opportunities and resources, these can be developed for empowerment. Valentine (1998) suggests that this has implications for children's nursing: 'For parents to be [empowered] to participate fully in their child's care new competencies may need to be learned or existing competencies developed' (1998, p. 24). Nurses need to help parents with this competency development. Empowerment involves first a process and then an outcome in family-centred care.

The outcome of empowerment

Power and control are key elements of an outcome of empowerment. Power in this context means that the family has the ability to be able to control the factors that are determining their lives. Social reality for families is likely to change when a child is sick, especially if continuing care is needed. This can create feelings of powerlessness and being out of control.

Power cannot be given to others; it has to be taken by individuals and communities (Rappaport, 1985); power is returned to people by a process of empowerment (Green and Raeburn, 1988). The outcome of this process is that individuals experience a change of power base (French, 1990). On our Practice Continuum, for example, care becomes parent-led as opposed to being nurse-led as families are empowered to take control of their changed social reality.

Within the practice of family-centred care nurses can use strategies to empower families. There will only be an outcome of empowerment, though, if the family takes power and control from nurses. This is 'power to' make decisions about their child's care, or 'power with' being able to give nursing or other care to their child. It does not mean power over others. Gibson (1995) found that the mothers of chronically-ill children were empowered when they had participatory competence in their children's care and were able to have their voices heard to participate in decision-making. This seems to agree with the notion of 'power to' and 'power with', described above.

Central to the notion of empowerment is the principle that individuals should be able to address problems that are important to them (Rappaport, 1985; Kalnins *et al.*, 1992). Families should be helped to identify problems that they perceive to be important and then helped by nurses to reach empowerment outcomes to deal with them. Nursing assessment is, therefore, important to prevent nurses making assumptions about family problems. Without this assessment, nurses could be disempowering families by only addressing problems diagnosed by nurses and not recognizing other problems that individual families may perceive as being important. Assessment is also necessary to identify cultural diversity within and between family units, which needs to be respected and valued if empowerment outcomes are to be achieved (RCN, 2000).

These empowerment outcomes are usually domain-specific. Wuest and Stern (1991) found, for example, that the families of children with middle-ear infections did not reach an outcome of effective management of care and remain empowered. This was because new situations would move them along a continuum towards more passive behaviours. The Practice Continuum for family-centred care in this book has the same underlying principles and recognizes that families are likely to move back and forth along the continuum depending on current situations. Wuest and Stern (1991) did find, though, with reference to empowerment outcomes, that 'over time families reported an increasing repertoire of management strategies, which they were able to use in different domains to achieve further empowerment outcomes.'

Families should therefore be helped by nurses to achieve empowerment outcomes through a process, with recognition that empowerment in one domain of the child's care is likely in time to lead to empowerment in another domain. In other words, empowerment is a regenerative process. So, for example, if parents first become competent in administering insulin to their child with newly-diagnosed diabetes, they are then more likely to want to re-enter the empowerment process to learn about other aspects of the child's care, such as altered dietary requirements.

Empowerment outcomes may be in either the physical, social or psychological domains. It seems that becoming empowered for many families could simply mean the development of a sense of psychological well-being. This promotes feelings of power and control, so that individuals no longer feel powerless. The family may then feel able to undertake aspects of physical care for their child and to participate socially with professionals in making decisions about care, functioning at the partnership level on the Practice Continuum. Families who subsequently reach the community or political level of empowerment will advocate to get material resources for their children, at the parent-led level on the Practice Continuum.

The process of empowerment

The process of empowerment is highly individual and it varies from one person to another (Lord and Farlow, 1990). It is recognized, though, that there are certain general factors that contribute to a personal empowerment process, and nurses need to be aware of these to be able to empower families. The work of Freire (1974) has been very influential in developing the concept of empowerment. Central to Freire's work was the notion of 'conscientization', which can be translated as the development of a critical consciousness. The purpose of critical consciousness-raising is to help people break free of false consciousness and to become aware of the reality of their situation. This is done in a four-stage process, according to Tones and Tilford (1994), which involves fostering reflection on aspects of personal reality, encouraging a search for and identifying the root causes of that reality, examining implications and then developing a plan of action to alter the reality. It seems that by using education to raise critical consciousness and awareness of reality, individuals or groups can be empowered to take action.

Kieffer (1984) found that an empowering process had four similar stages, an entry stage triggered by a specific incident, an advancement stage when mentor and peer relationships were important, a stage of incorporation in which self-development occurred, and a final stage of commitment in which participatory competence was achieved. Shields (1995) found that an internal sense of self emerges during an empowering process, which moves people to take action. This study also identified a salient theme of connectedness with the environment running throughout the empowering process, again suggesting that mentorship and peer relationships are important.

McWilliam *et al.* (1997) used an interactive process to empower participants in an action-research study. The process elements used built up on each other in a manner which enhanced the personal health of the participants in the study. The nurse and chronically-ill participants 'together evolved a caring relationship and an enhanced conscious awareness of life and health experiences' (McWilliam *et al.*, 1997, p. 111). During the process there was a building of trust and meaning, connecting, caring, mutual knowing and mutual creating. These strategies resulted in the acquisition of self-esteem, self-confidence and self-insight to enable the participants to make conscious choices about their lives. The individual's sense of control and empowerment was enhanced as a result of the relationship-building and heightened conscious awareness.

The relationship-building emphasized the significance of the reciprocity principle in an empowering process. The heightening of conscious awareness demonstrates again that the process has to commence with individuals reflecting on their personal reality, which may have changed because of a chronic illness. The emphasis in this study was on helping the participants to find out about themselves and their strengths and capabilities, to be able to empower themselves.

The study by Gibson (1995) about the process of empowerment in mothers of chronically-ill children had the opposite findings to the interactive nature of the process described by McWilliam *et al.* (1997). The empowering process was found to be largely intrapersonal by Gibson. Four stages emerged during this process, those of discovering reality, critical reflection, taking charge and holding on. The stages did not occur in a sequential order, they were interdependent and overlapping. The mothers in Gibson's (1995) study were motivated and sustained in the process of empowerment by the love they had for their children and the need to ensure that the best possible care was given. The frustrations encountered by the mothers when their usual ways of coping did not work was a predominant theme in the study:

> The frequency, intensity and duration of various frustrations evoked ongoing cycles of critical reflection which ultimately enabled the mothers to develop a sense of personal power and helped them to face reality. (Gibson, 1995, p. 1206).

Again the identification of critical reflection as a process element emphasizes the importance of facilitating it in an empowerment process, although the mothers in this study had to identify the need for it themselves. Paradoxically, a lack of interconnectedness between the mothers and the environment, which resulted in the frustrations, did support the process of empowerment. Shields (1995) identified connectedness as being important in a facilitated empowering process. There was some social support for the mothers, from families and nurses, but no facilitator 'to mentor them along their path to empowerment' (Gibson, 1995, p. 210). Children and families should have the right to be mentored along the path to empowerment especially during the advancement stage when according to Kieffer (1984) mentor relationships are important.

The rhetoric versus the reality of empowering families

There seems to be evidence that the rhetoric of empowerment is not always translated into the practice of family-centred care in reality. Kawik (1996), for example, found that parents were willing to participate in their children's care, but nurses were reluctant to relinquish their control of this care. Darbyshire (1994) identified that some nurses felt that parental participation was an alienating and exclusionary process that diminished the nurse's own role and deprived them of contact with parents and children. It is unlikely that these particular nurses would be using empowering strategies in practice.

This seems to happen despite evidence from both Fulton (1997) and Valentine (1998) that nurses possess the necessary theoretical knowledge to be able to empower children and families. The reason why they do not always do this in a family-centred approach to care seems to be twofold. One factor is that the key to empowerment is first the empowerment of nurses, according to Chevasse (1992), Fradd (1994) and Valentine (1998). The reality, however, is that nurses themselves are not always self-empowered (Baker, 1995), and so they are unable to facilitate a reciprocal social process within which children and families are helped to participate with competence, to take control over factors that affect their lives. In terms of the Practice Continuum offered in this book, families may be prevented from moving along the Continuum from nurse-led care towards family-led care, because of a lack of self-empowerment in nurses. Taking the reciprocity principle further, the environment within which family-centred care is implemented is often not empowering for either nurses or families. This may be the reason for nurses not always being able to provide the support to families that Gibson (1995) suggests is necessary for an empowering process to be efficacious.

The other reason for nurses not using theoretical knowledge about the concept of empowerment in practice seems to be a lack of knowledge about 'how' to empower in the practice of family-centred care. 'Simply espousing a philosophy of family-centered care does not ensure that the philosophy will be practiced' (Bruce and Ritchie, 1997, p. 220). Nurses do not always negotiate and share information with families or involve them in decision-making and care-planning in practice, because of a lack of skills in family dynamics, counselling, communication and interviewing (Bruce and Ritchie, 1997) It is the same with empowerment, an attribute of family-centred care. Valentine (1998) found that nurses were unable to empower families because they lacked the skills of teaching, assessing and supervising.

There has also been a tendency to look for weaknesses within the family unit, rather than finding strengths that need to be built upon to develop competencies and reach empowerment outcomes in a collaborative nurse–family relationship. Relationship-building is another key element of an empowering process which nurses seem to lack knowledge about in practice. Darbyshire (1994) found that there was an emphasis by nurses on the parents performing tasks as opposed to the development of life and health skills within empowering relationships. On our Practice Continuum, this may not always be inappropriate at the nurse-led levels, but pro-active planning is needed to enable families to develop these skills if care is to become parent-led for children with chronic conditions.

Coleman (1998) recommends the use of empowering models of nursing for family-centred care. The use of such models would prevent the *ad hoc* use of empowering strategies which can actually be disempowering to families because of a lack of planning and negotiation. A model used by Dunst and Trivette (1996) shows the relationship between three major components of the empowerment concept as in Table 5.1.

Coleman (1998) offers another empowering model for family-centred care as shown in Figure 5.1. This model suggests that

Table 5.1   A summary of Dunst and Trivette's (1996) empowerment model

Component 1   The model is underpinned by an empowerment ideology that believes everyone has the strengths, capabilities and the capacity to become competent. Therefore, during the process of empowerment, to maximize the likelihood of people becoming empowered, the emphasis should be on building strengths rather than correcting weaknesses

Component 2   involves participatory experiences. Opportunities are created for families to participate in care to strengthen their existing capabilities. The help-giving role of professionals involves active listening, empathy, compassion, warmth and caring, collaboration and shared decision-making with families

Component 3   is the achievement of empowering outcomes. Families develop the psychological attributes of self-efficacy beliefs, internal locus of controls and improved self-concepts, which result in empowerment outcomes

Empowerment = a regenerative process

If empowerment outcomes are reached at one stage of the process, families are encouraged to participate in the process again to achieve further empowerment outcomes

nurses need to be empowered themselves to be able to empower families in practice. Both these models can be used alongside the Practice Continuum proposed in this book. To be able to use these models in the practice of family-centred care, nurses need to know 'how' to empower. The next section aims to assist with this process by providing a toolkit for the empowerment of families.

How to empower families

Many families need help to develop or learn new competencies for empowerment (Rappaport, 1985; Valentine, 1998; Coleman, 1998), and a systematic approach is required for helping families to achieve empowerment outcomes. The nursing process provides the necessary systematic framework for this approach. The beliefs, values and ideologies of an empowering model of family-centred care (Dunst and Trivette, 1996; or Coleman, 1998) should be reflected in each of the four stages of the nursing process as shown in Table 5.2.

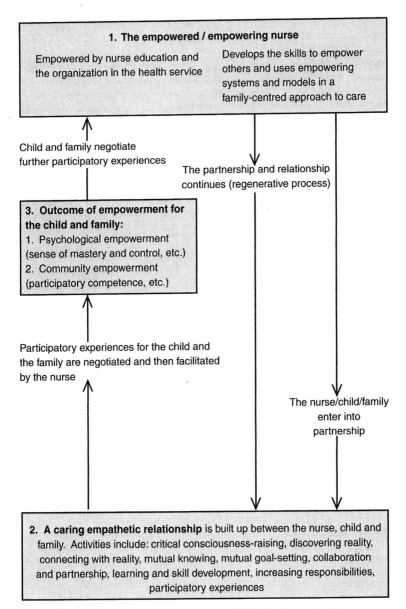

1. The empowered / empowering nurse

Empowered by nurse education and
the organization in the health service

Develops the skills to empower
others and uses empowering
systems and models in a
family-centred approach to care

Child and family negotiate
further participatory experiences

The partnership and relationship
continues (regenerative process)

**3. Outcome of empowerment for
the child and family:**
1. Psychological empowerment
(sense of mastery and control, etc.)
2. Community empowerment
(participatory competence, etc.)

Participatory experiences for the child and
the family are negotiated and then facilitated
by the nurse

The nurse/child/family
enter into
partnership

2. A caring empathetic relationship is built up between the nurse, child and
family. Activities include: critical consciousness-raising, discovering reality,
connecting with reality, mutual knowing, mutual goal-setting, collaboration
and partnership, learning and skill development, increasing responsibilities,
participatory experiences

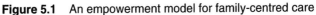

Figure 5.1 An empowerment model for family-centred care

Table 5.2   Empowering families using the nursing process

Assessment

During the assessment stage, nurses should be exploring family strengths and needs, rather than weaknesses, to facilitate the development of existing competencies. This is important to the promotion of self-efficacy beliefs in the family. If the family believes that they are able to take control over some domain of their child's care, a sense of psychological well-being develops. The family may then feel more able to learn new competencies for participation in other domains of their child's care

Family members are able to address problems that they themselves perceive as important, when needs are explored from their perspective. This avoids nurses making assumptions about the family's needs, which may actually be disempowering if the assessment is incorrect. Hartrick et al. (1994) offers a health-promoting family nursing assessment which emphasizes the importance of listening, sharing perceptions and participatory dialogue with the family during the assessment process

The assessment stage is the starting point for the relationship-building that is necessary during an empowering process. Reciprocity has been identified as a key to the achievement of empowerment outcomes (Coleman, 1998). Families need to be helped to develop competencies by empowered nurses or other professionals during an empowerment processes, although it is recognized that empowerment outcomes may also be achieved without help (Gibson, 1995)

Planning

The next stage of the process involves planning and negotiating participatory experiences with the family to enable them to become competent in negotiated domains of their child's care. To promote self-efficacy beliefs, which are fundamental to families being able to take power and control from professionals, goals need to be set which are initially short-term and achievable (Kemm and Close, 1995)

Implementation

During this stage of the nursing process, nurses should take on a helping role as described by Dunst and Trivette (1996). This involves helping families to undertake participatory experiences by providing them with technical knowledge, through giving information and/ or teaching them the necessary skills for caring for their sick children

Evaluation

The evaluation stage is necessary to see if the family has developed the negotiated competencies as a result of their participatory experiences. It is also to establish whether an empowerment outcome has been achieved with the family taking power and control from the professionals in relation to a particular domain of the child's care. Dependant on the evaluation, the nursing process cycle will be recommended, either to plan further participatory experiences to achieve the initial competency desired or to pursue the achievement of another competency. The empowerment model for family-centred care offered by Coleman (1998) suggests that families will be more likely to want to develop further competencies once success has been achieved in one domain of care

---

Some key activities for the development of family competencies have emerged from using the nursing process underpinned by an empowerment model. These key activities are:

- Relationship building.
- Facilitating participatory experiences.
- Helping families by information-giving (and teaching).

Nurses need to know how to use these familiar activities in a process of empowerment; they are discussed below with reference to empowerment and our Practice Continuum for family-centred care.

Relationship building

The building up of relationships between nurses and families is crucial to starting an empowerment process, since it is through these relationships that the families of sick children are able to develop a conscious awareness of their changed reality. Nurses need to listen and to develop trusting, meaningful relationships with families within which connecting and caring takes place (McWilliam *et al.*, 1997). This should result in nurses and families mutually knowing and mutually creating plans for the ongoing care of children together. The development of a sense of self-esteem, self-confidence and self-efficacy in family members is likely to be realized from relationship-building, and families with these feelings of psychological empowerment are more likely to want to take some personal control over their children's care and to negotiate participatory experiences with the nursing staff. To facilitate the building up of these relationships nurses need to utilize both their verbal and non-verbal communication skills and to apply them to the empowerment of families. This includes using negotiation skills, which are to be explored in Chapter 6.

Relationship building is perhaps easiest to do with the families of children who require continuing care. This is because building up a relationship takes time and there is more time available when there is continuing contact between families and nurses. Carter (2000) found that the levels to which community children's nurses were able to empower families were markedly different to the levels to which a hospital nurse could manage. Community children's nurses in Carter's study described their role as being to facilitate the family to the point where the nursing team could withdraw. Family-centred care in these cases would have become parent-led, in terms of our Practice Continuum.

It is important to recognize that these families may sometimes want respite from caring for their children. Families should be able to choose to participate at a different level on the Continuum for a period of time, after which respite is required. The relationships built up between families and nurses can be instrumental in bringing about recognition that movement back and forth along the Practice Continuum at certain times may be necessary. This is important, because without this recognition the families may actually become disempowered.

Some kind of relationship also needs to be built up with the families of children that are only in hospital for short periods of time. This is to empower them to participate in care at a negotiated nurse-led level on the Practice Continuum. Some families will want no involvement in care, only wishing to be present with their children for emotional support. However, quite often these families are disempowered because against their wishes they find themselves agreeing to be involved with their children's physical care. This may be due to nurses making the assumption that all families want to be involved in physically caring for their children. If time is taken to build up relationships, within which listening and an accurate assessment of family needs occurs, the appropriate level for family-centred care may be identified on the Practice Continuum and disempowerment avoided.

Conversely, other families may wish to participate in the nurse-led, physical care of their children. It is important, though, to still build up some kind of relationship within which these families feel they are able to negotiate the nature of the care in which they want to participate, otherwise nurses may make the incorrect assumption that parents want to participate in all care, which can again lead to families feeling out of control and powerless.

During the assessment process nurses should be using open-ended questions and encouraging the family to critically reflect to enable them to identify their own needs. Nurses need to actively listen to the family and check out what they are saying by paraphrasing and asking for clarification. Non-verbal communications, such as body posture and position, should also be used to convey to the families that the nurse is listening and to build up a relationship within which it is possible to say truthfully whether participation in care is desired or not. Nurses are then in a position to help with developing family competencies for empowerment at the appropriate level on the Practice Continuum.

Facilitating participatory experiences

It is necessary for families to have participatory experiences in relation to their child's care, and to be able to facilitate these experiences nurses require a clear understanding of what is meant by participation. The experience should also be a planned event, rather than the *ad hoc* disempowering affair which it appears to be on some occasions.

An attempt will now be made to bring some clarity to what constitutes a participatory experience, to promote empowerment as opposed to the disempowerment of families. These experiences may have physical, psychological or social dimensions as illustrated in Figure 5.2. They should be undertaken after negotiation with families. The focus needs to be on empowered nurses using their communication skills, technical skills and knowledge to participate with families, as opposed to families participating with nurses.

Physical participatory experiences are either about the performance of basic parenting tasks or doing nursing tasks. Darbyshire (1994) described basic parenting tasks as the care that mothers would normally give at home, such as hygiene care and feeding. The difference is that facilitated participatory experiences may be necessary to enable them to adapt their care to the changed situation in the hospital environment. For instance, it is not the same washing a child on traction in hospital as it would be at home in normal circumstances. Families require help and guidance during participatory experiences to become competent in performing these tasks. By the very nature of nursing tasks it can be deduced that families need participatory experiences to develop competencies. These tasks take a variety of forms, but may include giving injections, nebuliser therapy, inhaler administration and feeding by a naso-gastric tube. Nurses primarily tend to facilitate participatory experiences that involve the performance of physical tasks, and hence families are more likely to become

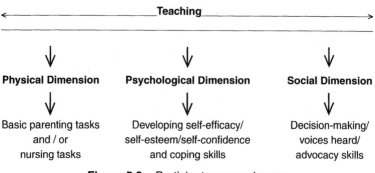

Figure 5.2 Participatory experiences

empowered in the physical dimension than the social and psychological dimensions. This may happen for a plethora of reasons, which include parents being used as a pair of hands, the reluctance of nurses to give up power and control and a lack of time or communication skills to develop psychosocial competencies. Families should be considered holistically, though, and to truly empower them participatory experiences in all dimensions need to be facilitated.

Social participatory experiences have the potential to empower families to have their voices heard by professionals and to actively participate in decision-making about their child's care. These experiences may also enable some families to develop the necessary competencies for advocating at a community level for resources and services for their children. These competencies can be developed to some extent through the aforementioned relationship-building, which has the potential to develop a sense of psychological well-being and coping skills. This development and the giving of information for informed decision-making are precursors to families being able to take action in the social domain.

An example of a participatory experience in the social domain could involve both the family and nurse being present during a discussion with members of the multidisciplinary team. The nurse's role is not only to support the family, but also to advocate for them and to ensure that they are able to ask questions and have their voices heard. In time, many families are likely to take power and control from the nurse and independently ensure that their voices are heard. Group membership of support groups has also been found to be empowering (Rissel, 1994), especially for children and families with a chronic condition. Nurses may facilitate this social participatory experience.

Participatory experiences in the psychological dimension will take place within the relationship-building that is needed for empowerment. The families will need some tangible positive feedback on their developing competencies in order to develop the feelings of self-efficacy, self-esteem and coping that are required to take power and control from nurses. To foster these feelings, short-term goals need to be set rather than long-term goals, in relation to a negotiated participatory experience. The development of a sense of psychological well-being may empower families to undertake participatory experiences in both physical and social domains.

Children should be exposed to empowering participatory experiences too. Those with such conditions as cystic fibrosis and diabetes will need to be taught how to perform physical nursing skills, so that they can take some control over their own care. Other children may be given choices related to play, to enable them to take some control over their situation. Children can be asked, 'what story would you like me to read to you?', or 'what toy would you like to play with?' Choices may also be given about nursing care, for example the child could take some control over wound care and the giving of medication (see Table 5.3).

Helping to empower families by information-giving

Information-giving is often seen as the key to empowerment. If families are given information, it can encourage them to undertake participatory experiences in their children's care which may lead to empowerment outcomes. Informed families are enabled to perform nursing care or alternatively adapt their usual parenting skills to care for their children, either in the hospital or the community. Information-giving may also help families to develop coping strategies, which will enable them to take some control over the situation in which they now find themselves with a sick child. It can lead to families being more likely to reach empowerment outcomes that involve them having their voices heard and participating in decision-making about their child's management

Table 5.3 Participatory experiences for children

The nature of the questions and the terminology will vary depending on the age of the child

Wound care
Choices could be given to the child, for example:

- When would you like me to change your dressing today – morning or afternoon?
- Where shall I do this – on your bed or in the treatment room?
- Do you want mummy to stay with you?
- Would you like mummy to read you a story whilst I do this?
- Do you want to help me clean your 'wound' today?

Giving medicine
A child has to take his medication. There is probably no choice about that, but there are other choices:

- Who do you want to give you your medicine – nurse or mummy?
- Would you like to swallow a tablet or drink some liquid?
- Do you want to take your medicine from a spoon or a medicine pot?
- What would you like to drink after you've taken your medicine?

---

and care. Informed families are in a better position to make choices and to give informed consent for interventions to be performed on their children.

Conversely, although nurses do act as information-givers in family-centred care, it could be suggested that an empowering approach to giving this information is not always used. Fleming (1992) argues, for example, that information-giving can be controlling, with the hidden agenda of producing good patients; the power base remains with the professionals and families are not empowered. Hartrick (1997) concurs with this view explaining that nurses predominantly use a model that teaches people about the nature of their health problems. This model assumes that the nurse is the expert and it pushes out family strengths and competencies. This kind of information-giving should be avoided because it does not produce empowered families (see Exercise 5.1). It is very important to value the family and to recognize their strengths in an empowering process.

A plethora of strategies and resources can be used to give information to families. Firstly, nurses and other professionals on a one-to-one basis can give verbal information to a family as part of

---

EXERCISE 5.1

Reflect on your clinical practice. Identify an incident when the giving of information did not help to empower a family. Analyse the incident and then list the reasons why information-giving was unsuccessful in helping to achieve empowerment outcomes in this incident. Your list may include the following reasons:

● Too much information was given.
● Insufficient information was given.
● Inappropriate information was given.
● Information sought by the family was not given.
● Information was given at the wrong time.
● The information needs of individual family members (which may be different) were not recognized.
● Information was given to the parents and did not involve the child at the appropriate developmental level.
● Inappropriate resources were used to help with the process of giving information.
● Information given may not have been understood, due to the use of jargon or language difficulties.

---

the relationship-building process; the nature of the information will vary depending on the family's individual needs. Teaching is integral to family-centred care and hence to empowerment and information-giving. Practical nursing skills may need to be taught to the family and also importantly, how to adapt their basic parenting skills for use in the hospital environment.

Skills teaching should be a planned event and the number of sessions it takes to work through the process described in Table 5.4 will be dependent upon the needs of individual families and the nature of the skill. Nurses may also be able to arrange for a family to meet other families that have children with the same problems. This facilitates a verbal sharing of information with peers, and it has already been identified that joining a more formal support group can be an empowering experience for families and it is certainly another forum for information-giving.

A second strategy for information-giving is the active use of literature to inform families. A plethora of leaflets have been produced in children's units as a response to the NHS's *The Patient's Charter: Services for Children and Young People* (DoH, 1996). These leaflets, which explain medical conditions, surgery, investigations

Table 5.4   Skill teaching

- Give information to the family so that they can fully understand the rationale for the care and why it is necessary. The most important things should be said first, stressed and repeated, so that they are remembered. Avoid saying too much at once and give specific precise information in a structured non-jargonized teaching session. Provide written information for the family to take away .Check to see if the family have understood the teaching (Ewles and Simnett, 1999)
- Demonstrate the skill to the family (as a whole skill or by breaking it into component parts)
- Provide opportunities for nurse and family members to perform the skill together to develop confidence and competency
- Assess and give feedback to the family members when they do perform the skill independently
- Family members become competent to practice the skill independently

---

and follow-up care, have the potential to inform families. Nurses should assess whether these leaflets are appropriate, though, for individual families and how they can be actively used as part of an information-giving process. Some families have been active themselves in the process of providing literature for information, and Willock and Grogan (1998) explained how parents and staff collaborated in the assessment of written information about renal diseases and then produced their own leaflets for use by families in the locality. This improved the families' understanding about the conditions and their involvement in this process empowered them to take a more active part in their own children's treatment. Books and posters are alternative written sources that could be used to inform families, but again their usefulness needs to be assessed.

Thirdly, more technical strategies could be utilized to inform, including videos, television programmes and computer learning packages. The Internet is another source of information that families may access to gain knowledge and understanding about their child's condition. In fact, the latest government policy (DoH, 1999) encourages them to do so, by using NHS Direct on-line. There are many other sources of information on the Internet though, some of which may be more credible than others. Nurses should respect the efforts of families to empower themselves by seeking information in this way and take time to sensitively discuss their findings with them, otherwise families may feel that their contribution to care is not being valued

Fourthly, information-giving to children may be facilitated through the use of play, which includes dolls, teddy bears and books. There is sometimes a tendency, though, to give information primarily to parents and not to involve children at an appropriate developmental level. It is important that children are included in an information-giving process, to explain what is expected of them in different situations. Story books have tended to give explanations about what health professionals will do to children with minimum reference to what is expected from them. Pre-admission preparation programmes for children have also been mainly about what other people will do to a child. Igoe (1993) proposes that to empower children, explanations about the role of others should not be eliminated, but they need to be balanced with stories and games that give the child a more active role. Wilson (1990) describes how young children with a chronic illness can become empowered through listening to stories about children that have an active responsible role in their own care. Responsibility is part of an empowering process, because it can increase both self-esteem and self-efficacy beliefs.

The interests of both nurses and family members may also affect the information-giving process in family-centred care. Habermas (1972) suggests that different people will have different interests, which determine their knowledge construction and their subsequent actions in practice. Hartrick (1997) applies this theory to the practice of nurses working with families, identifying that nurses with a technical interest will be motivated towards giving information to develop the practical skills of families; whilst other nurses with a more practical interest will find out about how every family member understands and experiences the child's condition. On the other hand, nurses with an emancipatory interest will focus on exploring with the family their capacity to live with the child's illness. It seems that nurses with practical and emancipatory interests would consider it very important to build up a relationship with the family for empowerment. These nurses would not only give information to the family, but also they would be very receptive to receiving information from the family, who are after all the experts on their own child.

The families themselves are also likely to have different interests, and an accurate nursing assessment is important to determine the information needs of individual families. Some families will be keen to learn technical skills for care, whilst others will want more time to exchange information with professionals in the process of family-centred care. It is becoming clear that information should be systematically given to families. This is essential if information-giving is truly to be the key to empowerment. In a study undertaken by Bailey and Caldwell (1997), it was found that families did not always recognize when nurses were giving them verbal discharge information, which was intended to prepare them for caring for their child at home; the families left hospital needing further information. This was partly due to nurses using an *ad hoc* approach to information-giving, rather than an empowering one that was planned and negotiated with the families (see Exercise 5.2).

A scenario will now be used to demonstrate, on our Practice Continuum, how a family may be empowered through information-giving and move back and forth along the continuum at different times, due to changing circumstances.

EXERCISE 5.2

During a nursing assessment, what data would you be seeking to determine the information needs of an individual family? Your answer may include the following:

- What information is needed/wanted by the family as a unit and as individuals?
- When is this information needed?
- How should the information be given to an individual family?
- What resources are available to help with information-giving?
- What information has the family to share with the nurses about their child and their social reality? (This is important during an empowering process, because parents are usually the expert on their child and can also provide information.)
- What are the family strengths?
- How would you evaluate whether appropriate information has been given, understood and empowerment outcomes achieved?

The assessment should facilitate a sharing of information between the nurse and family.

SCENARIO 5.1

James, who is 4 years old, is admitted to hospital with a diagnosis of asthma. He was always a wheezy baby and toddler and has been in hospital on two previous occasions. James is the first child of his parents, Tim and Jenny. He has a 2-year-old sister called Kirsty.

James's named nurse on the ward and the community children's nurse liaise to assess the family's needs for information. This liaison is important because on discharge the community nurse will be the person to maintain contact with the family. Continuity is helpful, especially in the early stages of the empowering process to prevent the family being disempowered by receiving contradictory messages from different healthcare professionals. During a process of critical consciousness raising, it is assessed that Tim and Jenny are very anxious about their ability to persuade James to use his prescribed inhalers. However, they feel comfortable holding and cuddling James when he has his nebuliser therapy. This is a family strength, and so is their desire to learn about his treatment. On reflection, it is apparent that they want to find out about the inhalers as soon as possible. Jenny is going to have to ensure James manages his inhalers at home on her own most of the time, because Tim works long hours. She believes that this may be difficult as James's sister Kirsty is quite a demanding 2-year-old. This is the family's social reality. So the family is interested in seeking information, which is of a technical orientation initially, to empower them.

Therefore, care is planned so that Tim and Jenny can be informed about the inhalers and how to use them. Initially, the nurses take the lead in helping James to use his inhalers. His parents are encouraged to observe how it is done and to ask questions about the procedure, to develop feelings of self-efficacy for empowerment. At this stage the family are at the *level of parental involvement* on the Practice Continuum. Assessment is ongoing and the nurses listen to the parents and negotiate with them about the right time for them to take the lead in helping James to use his inhalers. When his parents assume this role, the nurses observe and then give information back to Tim and Jenny on their efficacy in performing the procedure. The parents self-confidence increases as they develop the competencies to give James his inhalers safely and effectively. Positive feedback from the nurses on the performance of this technical skill helps to empower the parents. At this stage, Tim and Jenny have moved to the *level of parental participation* on the Practice Continuum.

James is also given information about how to use the inhalers, so that he has some control over his life in respect of his ongoing treatment. This is done through play activities with the involvement of the play specialist on the ward, who encourages James to handle the inhaler and pretend to give it to his favourite teddy bear. James is being empowered to take a role in the procedure. The play specialist also spends time playing with Kirsty, to distract and involve her when James and his parents are learning about the inhalers.

The initial parental need was for information on how to give James his inhaler. Once the parents are competent in actually being able to administer the inhaler to James, they have become empowered to do some of his care. It is important that they learn more about asthma and the action of the drugs that are given via the inhaler and other routes on occasions. At this stage family-centred care is still *nurse-led*. It is the nurses who take the initiative in giving this information to Tim and Jenny after assessing their readiness to receive it. The nurses give the information verbally to the parents, but also provide some leaflets for the parents to take away and read, to consolidate what has been explained verbally.

The information-giving process is commenced in hospital and continued on discharge by the community children's nurse. The community nurse develops a relationship with the family within which practical and emancipatory interests can be pursued in Hartricks' (1997) terms. The nurse can assess the understanding of individual family members about James's condition and explore their capacity to live with the child's illness (Hartrick, 1997). In other words, the nurse will not only be listening to the family, but will also be enabling them to have their voices heard and to be involved in decision-making about ongoing care, which are outcomes of empowerment. Family-centred care at this stage is now at the *level of a partnership* between the nurse and family on the Practice Continuum.

The family becomes expert in the management of James's asthma as he grows up. The information and the experience of living with asthma have empowered them to manage his condition; they understand the treatment and the need to avoid trigger factors that could precipitate an asthmatic attack. Family-centred care becomes largely *parent-led* on the Practice Continuum, apart from two occasions when James is readmitted to hospital. The family moved back along the Continuum temporarily to *nurse-led care* during these acute attacks that required hospitalization.

During adolescence, James starts to have more frequent asthmatic attacks, and when he is 15 years old he experiences another hospital admission. During the acute attack, family-centred care becomes *nurse-led*. His named nurse on the ward again liaises with a community children's nurse, who sees James and his family on the ward and later in the community after his discharge home. The community nurse assesses James carefully to discover if there are any particular reasons for his asthma being troublesome again. It is apparent that James has become embarrassed about using his inhalers, especially when he is out with his friends, and consequently he is not always using them when he should be. He also has a lot of pressure on him at the moment in relation to taking his GCSE examinations in the near future. The community nurse takes time to build up a trusting relationship with James, within which negotiation takes place to review the inhalers he is using and the times they need to be used. The intention is to enable him to use his inhalers at home, whenever possible, rather than when he is out with his friends. The community nurse also discusses some stress-relieving and coping strategies with James, to enable him to take some control over his forthcoming examinations. A *partnership* has again been entered into in terms of the Practice Continuum.

Within this trusting relationship, there will have been opportunities for the community nurse to give James further information about asthma and the importance of complying with treatment. James could have developed feelings of self-efficacy with this new information, resulting in him being more receptive to taking control of his asthma again. Family-centred care has the potential to become *parent-led* or in this case *adolescent-led* again on the Practice Continuum.

This scenario demonstrates how a family may ideally be empowered at different levels on the Practice Continuum, at different times.

In the clinical environment and society, though, there are often constraints and tensions which make it difficult to achieve empowerment outcomes. It is suggested that some reflective practice is now undertaken to identify your future learning needs about the empowerment of families (see Exercise 5.3).

Summary

This chapter has clarified the meaning of the concept of empowerment by exploring it as both an outcome and a process. It is suggested that empowerment is not always a reality in nursing practice and family-centred care, despite nurses apparently understanding it as a theoretical concept. It is recognized that there are many constraints and tensions within the practice environment that act as barriers to empowerment, but it is also apparent that nurses need to develop the necessary skills to make empowerment a reality for the families who want it. The chapter has also endeavoured to explain how to empower families through a process of relationship-building, facilitating participatory experiences, information-giving and teaching. It has provided a toolkit for empowering practice. Negotiation of care is part of an empowering process, and an exploration of approaches to negotiation within the context of family-centred care will now follow in Chapter 6.

EXERCISE 5.3

1. Reflect on a critical incident (that you were personally involved in) within which you thought a family was disempowered in hospital. Use the key stages of the empowerment process (relationship-building, participatory experiences and information giving/teaching) and the Practice Continuum in your analysis. What would you do differently in a similar situation?

2. Then reflect on another critical incident within which you were able to empower a family in some aspect of the child's care in hospital (acting on your learning from the previous reflection). How did you empower this family?

3. Choose a community experience with a family who you thought were empowered and undertaking parent-led family-centred care. Explain why you think they were empowered. Discuss with the community nurse her role in empowering this family. (Refer to the key stages of the empowerment process and the characteristics of empowerment outcomes).

4. Choose another community experience with a family who you thought were disempowered. Explain how you reached this conclusion. What was disempowering them? (Refer to empowerment processes and outcomes again in your answers).

References

Bailey, R. and Caldwell, C. (1997) 'Preparing Parents for Going Home', *Paediatric Nursing*, May, 9(4), pp. 15–7.

Baker, S. (1995) 'Family Centred Care: A Theory Practice Dilemma', *Paediatric Nursing*, July, 7(6), pp. 17–20.

Bruce, B. and Ritchie, J. (1997) 'Nurses' Practices and Perceptions of Family Centred Care', *Journal of Pediatric Nursing*, August, 12(4), pp. 214–22.

CCHS (1998) *Youth Matters: Evidence – Based Practice for the Care of Young People in Hospital* (London: Caring for children in the Health Services/Action for Sick Children).

Carter, B. (2000) 'Ways of Working: CCNs and Chronic Illness', *Journal of Child Health Care*, 4(2), Summer, pp. 66–72.

Chevasse, J. (1992) 'New Dimensions of Empowerment in Nursing and Challenges', *Journal Of Advanced Nursing*, 17(1), pp. 1–2.

Coleman, V. (1998) 'What is the Meaning of the Concept of Empowerment and Do Nurses Use It to Promote the Health of

Children with a Chronic Illness', unpublished Master's dissertation, Sheffield Hallam University.

Darbyshire, P. (1994) *Living with a Sick Child in Hospital: The Experiences of Parents and Nurses* (London: Chapman & Hall).

Department of Health (1996) *The Patient's Charter: Services for children and Young People* (London: HMSO).

Department of Health (1999) *Saving Lives: Our Healthier Nation* (London: Stationery Office).

Downie, R., Fyfe, C. and Tannahill, A. (1990) *Health Promotion Models and Values* (Oxford: Oxford University Press).

Dunst, C. and Trivette, C. (1996) 'Empowerment, Effective Helpgiving Practices and Family Centred Care', *Pediatric Nursing*, July/August, 22(4), pp. 334–7 and 343.

ENB. (2000) *Education in Focus: Strengthening Pre-Registration Nursing and Midwifery Education: Curriculum Guidance and Requirements* (London: English National Board).

Ewles, L. and Simnett, I. (1999) *Promoting Health: A Practical Guide*, Fourth Edition (London: Bailliere Tindall).

Fleming, V. (1992) 'Client Education: A Futuristic Outlook', *Journal of Advanced Nursing*, 17(2), pp. 158–63.

Fradd, E. (1994) 'Power to the People', *Paediatric Nursing*, 6(3), pp. 11–4.

Friere, P. (1974) *Education for Critical Consciousness* (London: Sheed & Ward).

French, J. (1990) 'Boundaries and Horizons, the Role of the Health Education within Health Promotion', *Health Education Journal*, 49(1), pp. 7–12.

Fulton, Y. (1997) 'Nurses Views on Empowerment: A Critical Social Theory Perspective', *Journal of Advanced Nursing*, 26, pp. 529–36.

Gibson, C. (1991) 'A Concept Analysis of Empowerment', *Journal of Advanced Nursing*, 16, pp. 354–61.

Gibson, C. (1995) 'The Process of Empowerment in Mothers of Chronically Ill Children', *Journal of Advanced Nursing*, 21, pp. 1201–10.

Green, I. and Raeburn, J. (1988) 'Health Promotion. What is it? What will it Become?', *Health Promotion*, 3(2), pp. 151–9.

Habermas, J. (Translated by Shapiro, J.) (1972) *Knowledge and Human Interest* (London: Heinemann).

Hartrick, G., Lindsay, A. E. and Hills, M. (1994) 'Family Nursing Assessment: Meeting the Challenge of Health Promotion', *Journal of Advanced Nursing*, 20, pp. 85–91.

Hartrick, G. (1997) 'Beyond a Service Model of Care: Health Promotion and the Enhancement of Family Capacity', *Journal of Family Nursing*, 3(1), pp. 57–69.

Hegar, R. and Hunzeker, J. (1988) 'Moving Towards Empowerment Based Practice in Public Child Welfare', *Social Work*, Nov/Dec, 499–502.

Igoe, J. (1993) 'Healthier Children Through Empowerment' in Wilson Barnett, J. and Macleod Clark, J. (eds), *Research in Health Promotion and Nursing* (London: Macmillan – now Palgrave), chapter 16, pp. 145–53.

Kalnins, I., McQueen, D., Blackett, K., Curtice, L. and Currie, C. (1992) 'Children, Empowerment and Health Promotion: Some New Directions in Research and Practice', *Health Promotion International*, 7(1), pp. 53–9.

Kawik, L. (1996) 'Nurses Attitudes and Perceptions of Parental Participation', *British Journal of Nursing*, 5(7), pp. 430–4.

Kemm, J. and Close, A. (1995) *Health Promotion: Theory and Practice* (London: Macmillan – now Palgrave).

Kieffer, C. H. (1984) 'Citizen Empowerment. A Developmental Perspective', *Prevention in Human Services*, 3(2/3), pp. 9–36.

Lord, J. and Farlow, D. (1990) 'A Study of Personal Empowerment; Implications for Health Promotion', *Health Promotion*, Fall, 2(2), pp. 2–8.

McWilliam, C., Stewart, M., Brown, J., McNair, S., Desai, K., Patterson, N., Del Maestro, N. and Pittman, B. (1997) 'Creating Empowering Meaning: An Interactive Process of Promoting Health with Chronically Older Canadians', *Health Promotion International*, 12(2), pp. 111–23.

Rappaport, J. (1985) 'The Power of Empowerment Language', *Social Policy*, 16, pp. 15–21.

Rissel, C. (1994) 'Empowerment: the Holy Grail of Health Promotion?' *Health Promotion International*, 9(1), pp. 39–46.

Robertson, A. and Minkler, M. (1994) 'New Health Promotion Movement: A Critical Examination', *Health Education Quarterly*, 21(3), pp. 295–312.

Rodwell, C. (1996) 'An Analysis of the Concept of Empowerment', *Journal of Advanced Nursing*, 23, pp. 305–13.

RCN (2000) 'Paediatric Nursing 2000: Draft Philosophy of Care', *Newslink for Nurses Working with Children and Young People*, Spring, (London: RCN).

Shields, L. (1995) 'Women's Experiences of the Meaning of Empowerment', *Qualitative Health Research*, 5(1), pp. 15–35.

Tones, K. (1997) 'Health Education as Empowerment', in M. Sidell, L. Jones, J. Katz and A. Peberdy (eds) (1997) *Debates and Dilemmas in Promoting Health: A Reader* (London: Open University, Macmillan – now Palgrave), chapter 4, pp. 33–42.

Tones, K. and Tilford, S. (1994) *Health Education: Effectiveness, Efficiency and Equity* Second Edition (London: Chapman & Hall).

Valentine, F. (1998) 'Empowerment: Family Centred Care', *Paediatric Nursing*, 10(1), pp. 24–7.

Willock, J. and Grogan, S. (1998) 'Involving Families in the Production of Patient Information Literature', *Professional Nurse*, March, 13(6), pp. 351–4.

Wilson, L. (1990) 'Storytelling for Children with a Chronic Illness', *Paediatric Nursing*, 6–7.

World Health Organization (1984) *Health Promotion: A Discussion Document on the Concepts and Principles* (Geneva: World Health Organization).

World Health Organization (1986) *Ottawa Charter for Health Promotion: An International Coference on Health Promotion* (Geneva: World Health Organization).

World Health Organization (1998) *Health 21: An Introduction to the Health for All Policy Framework for the WHO European Region*, European Health for All Series: No. 5 (Copenhagen: World Health Organization).

Wuest, J. and Stern, P. (1991) 'Empowerment in Primary Health Care: the Challenge for Nurses', *Qualitative Health Research*, 11(1), February, pp. 80–99.

6

Negotiation of Care

Lynda Smith

Introduction

The importance of developing a partnership with the child's parents and promoting the role of families in the care of their children has been stressed in the literature as well as being explicit government policy (Department of Health, 1991). Parents wish to participate in their children's care at a level of their own choosing, but what seems to be missing is either a willingness or the ability on the part of the nurse to always facilitate this process. It is therefore essential that children's nurses have the skills to negotiate with the child and family as this is seen as a fundamental element to the successful implementation of family-centred care.

This is essential if we are to give the quality of care and satisfaction children and their families need and want, and the use of communication skills is vital to implementing this family-focused care. Through negotiation involving collaboration and shared decision-making between all those involved in patient care, it is possible to provide the child and family with family-centred care which is the philosophy of children's nursing care.

This chapter will explore approaches to negotiation within the context of family-centred care in order to offer a framework for practice that will provide a meaningful dialogue between parents, healthcare professionals and children and young people. This collaboration between the relevant parties is aimed at achieving consensus in the relationship and provides a link to the Practice Continuum outlined in Chapter 2. Thus within the context of the

Practice Continuum, negotiation can take place at any point and is relevant to care that is nurse-led at one end of the scale to parent-led at the other. The approach taken will be clearly rooted in the practicalities of clinical practice and is applicable wherever that practice takes place, be that in the hospital or the community.

Negotiated care in nursing practice

Negotiation is a key element of nursing practice although Keatinge (1998) suggests that nurses often do not recognize the centrality of negotiation in their practice. Yet the call for nurses to negotiate care and roles with parents is a recurring theme in the family-centred care literature (Blower and Morgan, 2000; Neill, 1996; Casey, 1995). However, what has not been so clear is what constitutes negotiation in relation to family-centred care. Thus, if there is not clarity about what constitutes negotiation of care, how are staff and parents to become involved in this process and how will student nurses recognize that it is not happening and indeed needs to happen.

The *Concise Oxford Dictionary* (1990) defines 'negotiate' as to 'confer with others in order to reach a compromise or agreement', which would imply explicit dialogue that results in an agreed outcome. To achieve this in the context of family-centred care nurses, children and their families need to be involved in an open relationship whereby caring roles are established. Agreement is reached without any imposition or expectations being placed on each other (Newton, 2000). Additionally, understanding the context in which the negotiation takes place is important; there is no generic approach as each situation brings its own context-bound factors and issues.

Knafl and Dixon (1984) researching the participation of fathers summarized how nurses and parents might confer and reach an agreement. They felt that it was crucial that nurses explicitly discussed with parents how they would like to participate in their child's care and how the nurse and parents might work together in determining what their respective roles and levels of participation would be. In this example the relative position of each party is being made clear and provides part of the context in which negotiation may or may not take place. Thus negotiation does not take place in a vacuum, and it is necessary to consider the relative positions of the nurse and the family in the context of provision of care and the importance thereof of the balance of power and control within the relationship (Callery and Smith, 1991). These elements and others that may affect successfully negotiated care will now be considered.

Negotiation failure

Whilst it is possible to articulate the ideal collaborative relationship, research studies would suggest it is easier to describe the elements of successfully negotiated care than to achieve it. Studies that have identified negotiation as a feature of parental participation have identified the need for planned negotiation with parents and the reasons why nurses fail to negotiate and pay lip-service to the concept (Kawik, 1996; Dearmun, 1992; Evans, 1994). Thus factors that influence parents' and nurses' abilities to negotiate are identified, such as territory (environment) stress/anxiety of the parents, power and control of the nurses and the skills of negotiation.

Power and control

Potentially the balance of power and the ability to control rests clearly with the nurse. Essentially parents are entering the nurse's domain as she has the advantage of familiarity with the environment and belongs there by virtue of her role within the organization. Conversely, the parents are visitors in an unfamiliar area with the added vulnerability of being concerned for their child's well-being. Coping with the stressors of hospitalization, it is easy to see that parents may feel unsure of their role and ill at ease performing even the basic parenting tasks.

Implicit in the notion of bringing your child to hospital is that that action represents a handing over of control to the professional, almost an unspoken agreement that parents want staff to care for their child (Baker, 1995; Callery and Smith, 1991). Thus differing perceptions may lead to negotiation failures as parents feel disempowered and nurses feel the need to protect their role as the knowledgeable expert.

Part of negotiated care is the ability of the parents to feel empowered to make informed choices and decisions; this has been discussed in detail in Chapter 5. However, in the context of negotiated care and issues of control, where the nurse is reluctant to relinquish control, she may become the 'gatekeeper' of the knowledge parents need in order to make informed decisions and also to sharing with and teaching parents the relevant skills to become more actively involved in the care of their child. Essentially the nurse controls information and the potential is then for a power struggle between nurses and parents. As power and control are both factors which influence the negotiation process, there is a need to promote empowerment to facilitate this process (Trnobranski, 1994). It is important, therefore, to utilize the approaches to facilitating empowerment in practice identified in Chapter 5 to support the development of negotiation skills highlighted in this chapter.

Control can also be seen from the parents' perspective as being a coping strategy. In Evan's (1994) study participating in their child's care gave the mothers a feeling of control and this was fundamental to their coping strategies. This involved negotiating with professionals to reach a state of equilibrium; however this did not negate the potential for power struggles between the mothers and nursing staff. These findings, though, are not generalizable as the sample were five mothers of chronically-ill children and related to a specific programme of teaching to aid their participation in administering intravenous antibiotics.

Negotiation or expectation?

Where parents actively contribute to the care of their child and are welcomed into the clinical area, their role is not always clear due to a failure to negotiate care with them. Three studies in particular highlight the assumptions made by nurses with regards to parental involvement in care. Kawik (1996) surveying nurses and parents with regards to their perceptions of participation and partnership, found that nurses often assumed that parents would like to be involved in the nursing care yet did not always negotiate the extent of that care. They were unwilling to relinquish control and she also found little evidence of partnership;

instances of parental participation occured on an *ad hoc* basis rather than as a result of planned negotiation in care.

Equally, Neill (1996) examining the experiences of participation in the care of children and factors that facilitate or inhibit this process supports this view. Her results showed that parents felt that nursing staff assumed they would look after their child if they were present with their child in hospital. Alongside this was a feeling of being left to get on with it. Parents want to be able to negotiate with nursing staff to establish their own role and that of the nursing staff and thereby have some control over the extent of their involvement. The only example of this type of negotiation was when a nurse merely asked the mother if she wanted to look after her child.

Dearmun (1992) included student nurses in her study researching perceptions of parental participation. Commenting on the extent that parents were expected to contribute to care, it was clear from both qualified staff and student nurse perceptions that involvement by parents was taken for granted and, as with the other studies highlighted, it was assumed when parents were present they would take over.

These studies give an insight into the nature of the relationships that exist between nurses and parents and do not appear reflective of those where positive negotiation can flourish. That is, those based on mutual understanding of parent and nursing roles underpinned by collaborative, open, honest relationships. Yet the ideas and beliefs about family-centred care put forward by nurses in Baker's (1995) study reflect those espoused by the literature. However, the interviews revealed that the nurses did not always transfer the concepts into practice.

Stress and anxiety

There are clearly communication issues to be addressed. However, it may be that whilst parent's perceptions are that they are left to get on with it, they have misinterpreted the nurse's intention. Hospitalization is a very stressful experience, for parents as well as children, hence the importance of utilizing a framework for practice that involves the ways in which these messages are communicated.

Positive negotiation

In contrast, the experience of community children's nurses is seen as more positive and that partnerships are more easily facilitated in the community (Gould, 1996). Taylor (2000), comparing partnerships in the community and hospital, felt that the difference in experience was due to the balance of power being reversed, as the nurse was now the visitor. Parents also felt more informed about their child's progress which increased confidence in caring for their child and their ability to input into the relationship with the nurse. The ongoing relationship between community children's nurses and families enhanced the communication process whereas in hospital parents had to relate to a variety of people. These differences enable the community children's nurse to facilitate the philosophy that underpins paediatric nursing, so that parents in the community meet the ongoing care needs of their children with support from the community nurses (Sidey, 1990). Much of the research in negotiating care with families has taken place in the hospital setting, but given the positive experience of the community nurse it may well be valuable to look more closely at this area of practice to distil a framework that may be transferable between settings and clearly root negotiation and partnerships in children's nursing practice.

Negotiation skills

If negotiation is clearly not happening with parents, how can this be facilitated, how can nurses develop these skills? This is important as it may be difficult for student nurses, in the absence of appropriate role models, to develop these skills in clinical practice and thus once qualified they do not feel equipped to fulfil this role either. Hence the cycle is repeated. One study by Eddy and Schermer (1999) highlighted the value of shadowing as a strategy to strengthen the negotiation style of nursing students, however this is dependent on having role models to shadow with the necessary skills.

Callery and Smith (1991) in an exploratory study of role negotiation between nurses and the parents of hospitalized children questioned whether negotiation takes place at all. Using a critical-incident technique, 64 nurses described their responses to their perception that a parent wants to increase or decrease involvement in their child's care. Nurses' responses were categorized into categories of encouragement, advice and negotiation. The study was limited by the level of inter-rater reliability, particularly in the category of negotiation. However, the results were suggestive of significant association between the category of response and the grade of staff. The more senior the staff the more the response was one of negotiation. Implications for nurse education were suggested, in particular preparation in the skills of negotiation are required if nurses are to negotiate effectively with parents.

Thus where there is a willingness to negotiate the barrier seems to be the nurses' ability to transpose the concept into day-to-day practice. The second part of this chapter offers a framework that is practical and geared towards incorporation of the key elements of negotiated care into everyday working practice, both for students and practitioners.

Negotiation frameworks and guidelines for practice

Negotiation is often thought of in terms of trade union agreements and hostage-type situations and there will be a body of literature that addresses communication in these instances. However, negotiation frameworks outlined in this section have been selected because they specifically relate to caring for children and their families, though there will be some commonality in terms of principles between any of the approaches to negotiation.

The negotiating model (Dale, 1996)

Dale (1996) has written comprehensively about partnership, particularly in relation to working with families of children with special needs, and has devised the Negotiating Model. This she puts forward as a model of partnership, developed from the premise that negotiation is a key transaction for partnership to work (see Table 6.1).

Table 6.1 Elements of Dale's (1996) negotiating model

The key elements of this model include the following:

- Parents and professionals have separate and potentially highly valuable contributions to offer
- Each person may therefore require the contribution of the other
- Each come to the encounter with separate or different perspectives of their situations
- The professional has a responsibility to provide a service and bridge the gap between the different perspectives by learning about the parent's perspective
- Two-way dialogue and negotiation occurs, with each partner bringing their own perspective to assist in the decision-making
- Negotiation can lead to two outcomes: shared understanding and consensus, or lack of shared understanding and dissent
- The partnership relationship may be a cyclical process, which shifts between agreement and disagreement
- In extreme disagreement the partnership may be temporarily or permanently inoperative

---

The approach taken by Dale seems to be from the standpoint of identifying issues of mutual concern and through negotiation resolving these differences. This is clear from the definition:

> a working relationship where partners use negotiation and joint decision making and resolve differences of opinion and disagreement, in order to reach some kind of shared perspective or jointly agreed decision on issues of mutual concern. (Dale, 1996, p. 56)

In day-to-day nursing practice negotiation of care might include this perspective, but very often conflict and disagreement has arisen as a result of non-negotiation of roles predominantly in the hospital setting. Negotiation therefore needs to take place from the outset at a very basic level and develops as the relationship develops. Thus developing the skill in practice is essential to the children's nurse.

Guidelines for the negotiation of parental participation in care

In developing the skills of negotiation, support from guidelines for practice are valuable to the nurse in developing the role and

Table 6.2   Guidelines for negotiation abridged from Ireland (1993)

1. Specific guidelines/standards in relation to the role of the parent. Early communication and documentation of the parents' role in care is essential and should be incorporated into the nursing care plan
2. Each negotiation needs to start with consideration of the meaning that the child's hospitalisation has for the family and exploration of their needs and goals
3. There needs to be a shared understanding of the concept by everyone in the healthcare team (thus there will be no variation between shifts and individual nurses)
4. Time and information need to be available to enable parents to be involved
5. Parents need support, hence facilities are important for them also, as is support for renegotiation of their role (this needs to be done on a daily basis and accurately documented)
6. There is a need to accept variations in coping (relates to changes in a child's condition, treatment and family life)

providing a baseline approach for all staff to follow. An example of a set of guidelines has been produced by Ireland (1993), and an abridged version is listed in Table 6.2.

Incorporating these guidelines into a clearly identifiable framework for practice should promote negotiation in practice. With this in mind, the final section of this chapter provides a step-by-step guide to negotiation in children's nursing practice. This has been developed by the author as a practical way to teach the skill in the classroom setting. Personal experience in this field with student nurses found that whilst student nurses were able to identify the need for and the importance of negotiated care, what they also needed was the know-how to put it into their practice. Their exposure to the skill in practice was variable and they clearly needed to be able to link together the theory and the practice in a way that made sense and was 'doable' within the constraints experienced in busy clinical areas. The framework has been developed from the phases of bargaining by Gourlay (1987) and linked explicitly to the nursing process as this is a familiar concept to all nurses. In utilizing this framework, the nurse can also draw upon the guidelines identified by Ireland and the negotiation model provided by Dale.

Gourlay (1987) advocates negotiation as a way of bringing about an agreement. Negotiations are essentially a voluntary relationship between two parties with one person trying to persuade another to accept his point of view. If successful, both parties feel that their needs have been satisfied and are committed to implementing the decision. Thus negotiations are about meeting people's needs:

> Negotiations are interpersonal relationships in which communications play a vital role. For there to be an outcome in which both parties win, it is essential that each is able to communicate clearly with the other. (Gourlay, 1987, p. 25)

In utilising this step-by-step approach to negotiation the practitioner needs to use all the basic skills and approaches to communication they have previously developed. These include verbal, non-verbal and written skills. Applying those skills specifically to the negotiation process will remove barriers to successful communication and facilitate the development of a working partnership with the child and family.

It is timely at this point to re-emphasize the value of the communication framework LEARN (Berlin and Fowkes, 1983), highlighted in Chapter 2, which can be utilized as part of the communication and collaboration between nurse and family. The acronym identifies the following:

L – Listen empathetically and with understanding to the family's perception of the situation
E – Explain your perception of the situation
A – Acknowledge and discuss the similarities as well as differences between the two perceptions
R – Recommend interventions
N – Negotiate an agreement on the interventions

Phases in the negotiation process

1. *Structuring expectations*

   ● Identifies boundaries and minimizes the gap between the hopes of both parties.

   For example, the guidelines and philosophy of the unit/ward should have been shared in advance (obviously they need to contain elements of and reference to the valuing of parental involvement in care to the level with which they wish to be involved) Parents will therefore have some idea about the potential for involvement and the fact that there will be explicit dialogue about it at a suitable point.

2. *Discovering the other's needs (ASSESS)*

   - You should be concentrating on the needs and requirements of others – what they want from the negotiation rather than what you want.
   - Use open-ended questions – how, why, where, when, what?
   - Remember, don't forget the value of listening, silence, paraphrasing.

   It is timely here to remember the barriers to successful communications in the negotiating process; these are outlined following the five phases of the negotiating process.

3. *Moving towards settlement (PLAN)*
   The parties need to:

   - Be empowered to make decisions – refer to the previous chapter on empowerment and identify what this means in terms of empowering the nurse as well as empowering the parents.
   - Understand what is on offer, this will avoid some of the pitfalls identified by the research into family-centred care.
   - Identify any points that are not acceptable, remember communication needs to be open and honest.
   - Record points made, that is the agreements, this is important to facilitate continuity of the agreement to all involved parties and thus avoid changes in management between different nurses and different shifts.

4. *Achieving agreement (IMPLEMENT)*

   - Package gets wrapped up; for example in nursing practice the care plan is produced. Points to consider include how is the negotiated care documented, by whom, and when? Is there scope for written as well as verbal comments by parents?
   - Summarize agreements made, ensuring both parties understand.

- Don't leave loose ends, be clear about responsibility and accountability, these issues are discussed in Chapter 8.

5. *Reviewing the agreement (EVALUATE)*
   Build in time when agreements can be reviewed – in nursing this would be evaluation/review

   - It is not always possible to know how agreements will work out in practice.

   By creating a review mechanism you allow both parties to develop confidence in taking a risk with the agreement; that is, if it doesn't work out, change it

What may negatively influence this process?

Negotiations are interpersonal relationships in which communication plays a vital role. However, sometimes the message gets distorted during the transmission and reception phases. If we are able to identify the causes of these distortions we should be able to improve the quality of the communication and hence in this instance the negotiated care. Gourlay (1987) identifies two main factors that cause distortion of communication. 'Filters' may be seen as a psychological block which then distorts what another person is saying, and 'double messages' which occur when more than one message is being sent at a time.

Filters can relate to assumptions, preconceptions and defensiveness, each of which will be considered in terms of its potential to effect negotiated care.

- *Assumptions:* we often assume that we know what the objectives and needs of the other party are. Thus from the literature reviewed so far, it is clearly often assumed that because parents are present they will want to be involved in care in a way the nurse expects they should be. To some extent this is often a reflection of the nurse's own values and beliefs of parenting as if they themselves were in that position. By not acknowledging the parents' own reference frame and finding out their needs and wishes a communication block is in place and therefore you may not hear what they are really saying to you.

- *Preconceptions*: we make inferences from the information that we have. In reflecting on practice experience, first impressions often set the tone for subsequent communications. Do we communicate differently with families from 'professional/ middle-class' backgrounds as opposed to families from other socioeconomic backgrounds? We may assume that more articulate families are able to traverse the healthcare system more easily than other families, and vice versa. This may also lead to preconceptions about the degree of their involvement. Either way, we may not hear the messages being sent accurately.
- *Defensiveness*: we protect ourselves from criticism by ascribing blame or faults in our own behaviour or actions to others. In this situation we need to be aware of our own limitations and not ascribe failures in the communication process solely to the parents. Sometimes the families' quest for understanding and information about their child and the nature of the problems being experienced can leave the nurse feeling challenged as though his/her role as an expert is being questioned. This can lead to a defensive reaction, exemplified by the 'nurse knows best' approach; rather, the nurse needs to remember the difference between being an expert in his/her chosen field, and parents as experts in relation to their child. Communication skills have to be learnt and developed with experience. By understanding ourselves in the context of our own personal development it is possible to move forward, where necessary be open to criticism and improve our skills significantly.

Double messages may send out a covert communication which is actually the opposite of what is being said. In relation to negotiated family-centred care we need to be sure that we say what we mean and mean what we say. Thus if we believe in negotiated care on the basis that parents make informed choices and decisions about the extent of their involvement in their child's care, then we have to be sure that that is the only message that we are sending out. It is easy for parents to feel guilty if they for many reasons cannot be with their child or participate as actively in their child's care as other parents. Parents' perceptions of their experiences in hospital with their child suggest they can feel guilty leaving their child for a short break (Darbyshire, 1994). This can be avoided if we avoid sending out double messages. Remember that communication is more than a verbal process, non-verbal communication can belie what we are saying.

What positive attributes may positively influence this process?

Effective communication is the key to successfully negotiated care. The framework provides a step-by-step process, but to achieve a successful outcome it has to be underpinned by the use of communication skills. Being a skilled listener is essential, as identified by the LEARN framework, in order to hear what the other party is saying. This is not as easy as it sounds and takes practice, although communication exercises can help fine-tune skills.

An open approach is frequently referred to but not always followed through in practice. In nursing, sharing of information is an example of this and links with earlier discussions on power and control and empowerment. Positive non-verbal approaches are important as they demonstrate an interest in what the other party has to say. The utilization of skills previously learnt such as making eye contact and sitting forward is important. It is also important to clarify the communication that has taken place, to reduces the potential for communication distortion. Paraphrase what the other party has said, and repeat back what you think they've said. By using this facilitative style you can clarify the needs of the child/family and make sure there are no loose ends.

Being able to use effective communication skills is a developmental process, and the relevance of this to family-centred care can be seen in Chapter 7 where the focus is on learning to practice such care. Experiential reflective learning is promoted as building blocks through which student nurses will develop their skills for practice at pre-registration and beyond. The following practice exercises are designed to to be carried out over a period of time to facilitate reflection on one's own personal development and, where relevant, to identify the broader needs of the clinical area in which you work.

EXERCISE 6.1

Select a recent patient-care scenario where you had significant involvement with the child and family, preferably one where you were involved in the initial admission/referral. Reflect in detail from admission to discharge the involvement in care by the family.

Using the negotiation guidelines and the phases in the negotiation process analyse the extent to which the child's care was negotiated with the family. Identify positive and negative aspects, in particular those areas you need to develop further to enhance your personal skills.

Additionally identify areas that may need to be developed as a ward, unit or team, for example written communication. At a later point you may wish to think about how you might overcome any barriers to development in this area. This may involve a review of approaches to change management, if this was an area you were interested in pursuing.

EXERCISE 6.2

Having reflected on a recent practice scenario, for the next child and family you admit or have referred to you, utilize the negotiation process. Reflection on and during practice will enable you to determine the extent to which you feel negotiation is taking place. Again identify those aspects that went well and those that were not as successful. If unsuccessful why? Where possible identify how can this be overcome. Remember practice is essential in developing communication skills, and confidence develops with experience.

EXERCISE 6.3

Using the same approach, reflect on different types of admissions/referrals; for example short-stay and longer-stay admissions, or regular patients. Does it make any difference to using the process?

EXERCISE 6.4

Where you were involved with families in situations where there were issues of concern to be resolved, for example the family and practitioner had differing perspectives on an issue, did the negotiation process facilitate this? If not, why not? were additional strategies needed to support the process?

Summary

Negotiated care in children's nursing practice is a key element of family-centred care. Facilitating the skill in practice has been problematic and nurses' failure to negotiate with families has been seen largely as a reluctance to relinquish power and control and embrace families as partners in care. Additionally, the ability of nurses to negotiate has also been questioned and the need for skills in this area identified.

An essential part of this process is the utilization of appropriate and effective communication skills. Models and guidelines that facilitate negotiated care in paediatric settings are available but underutilized. The second part of this chapter therefore focused on creating a framework for student nurses and practitioners to develop and utilize in practice. By creating a framework for negotiation linked to a systematic approach to care, a concept familiar to all nurses, it is hoped this will support the implementation of negotiated care in children's nursing practice. Chapter 7 will continue this process by looking at how learning family-centred care in practice can be facilitated through experiential, reflective approaches.

References

Allen E. (ed.) (1990) *The Concise Oxford Dictionary of Current English*, 8th edn (Oxford: Clarendon Press).

Baker, S. (1995) 'Family Centred Care: A Theory Practice Dilemma', *Paediatric Nursing*, 7(6), pp. 17–20.

Berlin E. A. and Fowkes W. C. (1983) 'A Teaching Framework for Cross-Cultural Health Care', *Western Journal of Medicine*, 139(6), pp. 934–38

Blower, K. and Morgan, E. (2000) 'Great Expectations? Parental Participation in Care', *Journal of Child Health Care* 4(2), pp. 60–5.

Callery, P. and Smith, L. (1991) 'A Study of Role Negotiation Between Nurses and the Parents of Hospitalised Children', *Journal of Advanced Nursing*, 16, pp. 772–81.

Casey, A. (1995) 'Partnership Nursing: Influences on Involvement of Informal Carers', *Journal of Advanced Nursing*, 22, pp. 1058–62.

Dale, N. (1996) *Working with Families of Children with Special Needs, Partnership and Practice* (London: Routledge).

Darbyshire, P. (1994) *Living with a Sick Child in Hospital: The Experiences of Parents and Nurses* (London: Chapman & Hall).

Dearmun, A. (1992) 'Perceptions of Parental Participation', *Paediatric Nursing*, 4(7), pp. 6–9

Department of Health (1991) *Welfare of Children and Young People in Hospital* (London: HMSO).

Eddy, M. E. and Schermer, J. (1999) 'Shadowing: A strategy to Strengthen the Negotiating Style of Baccalureate Nursing Students', *Journal of Nursing Education*, 38(8), pp. 364–7.

Evans, M. (1994) 'An Investigation into the Feasibility of Parental Participation in the Nursing Care of their Children', *Journal of Advanced Nursing*, 20, pp. 447–82.

Gould, C. (1996) 'Multiple Partnerships in the Community', *Paediatric Nursing*, 8(8), pp. 27–31.

Gourlay, R. (1987) *Negotiations for Managers Health Services Manpower Review* University of Keele

Ireland, L. (1993) 'The Involvement of Parents in Self-Care Practices', in E. A. Glasper and A. Tucker (eds), *Advances in Child Health Nursing* (Harrow: Scutari Press), chapter 15, pp. 195–203.

Fletcher, K. (1998) *Negotiation for Health and Social Services Professionals* (London: Jessica Kingsley).

Kawik, L. (1996) 'Nurses and Parents' Perceptions of Participation and Partnership in Caring for a Hospitalized Child', *British Journal of Nursing*, 5(7), pp. 430–4.

Keatinge, D. (1998) Negotiated Care... Fundamental to Nursing Practice', *Journal of The Royal College of Nursing*, Australia, 5 (1) 36–42

Knafl, K. A. and Dixon D. M. (1984) 'The Participation of Fathers in their Child's Hospitalisation', *Issues in Comprehensive Pediatric Nursing*, 7(4–5), pp. 269–281.

Neill, S. (1996) 'Parent Participation', *British Journal of Nursing*, 5(2), pp. 110–7.

Newton, M. S. (2000) 'Family Centred Care: Current Realities in Parent Participation', *Pediatric Nursing*, 26(2), pp. 164–8.

Sidey, A. (1990) 'Co-operation in Care (Family Centred Care for the Child with Cystic Fibrosis at Home)', *Paediatric Nursing*, 2(3), pp. 10–12.

Taylor, J. (2000) 'Partnership in the Community and Hospital: A Comparison', *Paediatric Nursing*, 12(5), pp. 28–30.

Trnobranski, P. H. (1994) 'Nurse-Patient Negotiation: Assumption or Reality', *Journal of Advanced Nursing*, 19(4), pp. 733–7.

7

Learning to Practice Family-Centred Care

Sue Ford

Introduction

The challenges for nurse education that have been identified in previous chapters have revolved around translating the theory of family-centred care into the practice of individual nurses. This is no great surprise to anyone involved in nurse education; the theory–practice relationship within nursing has been heavily criticized for many years. Hislop *et al.* (1996) suggest that a situation exists in nurse education in which theoretical knowledge is neither accessible nor appropriate in practice. Eraut *et al.* (1995) agree that nursing theory is often regarded by nursing students as knowledge they cannot use:

> Not necessarily irrelevant to practice, but irrelevant to current practice.Theory can be used to evaluate current practice, but it is best done in the safety of an essay, rather than risk upsetting qualified staff in their placements. (Eraut *et al.*, 1995, p. 9)

Despite an emphasis in nurse education on comforting, teaching and maintaining therapeutic relationships with families (Pounds, 1989), there is evidence to suggest that students are not always learning these principles. There is a dichotomy for the student in practice, in that whilst there is a continuing expectation that nurses provide holistic care there is a greater demand placed upon them in terms of technical care (UKCC, 1999). Thus, as

Greenwood (1993) claims, in practice students learn that 'real' nursing is all about technical, medically evolved procedures and nursing care is simply getting through the workload of mundane activities. When learner nurses observe this behaviour in the practice setting they are subject to a process of professional socialization in order to be accepted by their nursing teams. French (1992) claims that the result is a preregistration preparation that is not an educational experience but instead produces practitioners who are uncritical replicators of existing nursing practice.

Gray and Smith (1999), in their longitudinal study of the professional socialization of diploma nursing students, identified the mentor as the linchpin of the student's experience. There are, of course, a great many nurses who maintain extremely high standards of care and who act as excellent role models for students. Schools of nursing, however, cannot guarantee that it will be such practitioners who will be the chief influence on their student nurses, and the general lack of nurse lecturers with an active practice role can result in academic staff lacking credibility with students.

Nurse education is under pressure to produce practitioners able to enter the workforce with the relevant skills and levels of preparedness for practice (UKCC, 1999). The key is to examine practice as the most influential learning environment, and then to draw out how educational efforts can be best directed to make learning meaningful and applicable.

The realities of practice

When they are asked why family-centred care so often fails to be evident in practice, students, qualified nurses and even families often give responses focused on the problems of the practice environment. Lack of time to talk with families, busy ward environments, lack of resources to care for parents, fast turnover of patients and staff shortages feature prominently in any discussion about implementing family-centred care. The use of support staff to carry out many of the nursing interventions described as 'basic' nursing skills leads to the qualified staff spending less time, less often with each of the families in their care. Add to this not only the element of confusion surrounding definitions and terms used, but also the whole issue of authority and responsibility when sharing care with families, and the principles learned in the safety and calm of the classroom can seem a dim and distant distraction.

A major difficulty for learners in their practice placements is making sense of broad concepts and critically discussing their experiences. The unstructured, unpredictable nature of the practice setting has been found to lead to qualified staff using habitual, standardized modes of patient care given in a routinized manner in order to maintain some measure of control and accountability (Johns, 2000; Procter, 1989). In such environments and with staff developing such coping strategies, discussion and analysis of care with the student who is following the mentor around is not likely to be a priority. The aim of this chapter is to describe a developmental process in which learners can progress through the levels of understanding of family-centred care, from practising fundamental communication skills, through to reflecting on their own practice. It is aimed at the students themselves but may also be useful to the practitioners and teachers who are working with them to develop their skills in this area. The process of learning about family-centred care in the practice setting relies upon gradually building the next layer of knowledge on the foundations of practising the previous one. This is likely to continue way beyond student years into post-registration professional development. This, then, is part of lifelong learning and rightly so. Much attention has already been paid in previous chapters to the higher levels of knowledge underpinning family-centred care; here it is important to address the early stages of development at the very beginning of the learning process. Once this has been addressed, the more complex levels of understanding will become more accessible and applicable to personal practice.

Getting started

Family-centred care, as evidenced in previous chapters, has a significant knowledge base and can be studied using a variety of conceptual and theoretical frameworks. These require some degree of determination to fully appreciate, and novice nurses may find it difficult to explain their actions in such terms. Education is a developmental process; learning needs to be facilitated along a developmental continuum that aligns understanding with experience.

A major problem experienced by junior students with regard to family-centred care is that they lack the experience to enable them to make sense of the theory. Ausubel *et al.* (1978) claim that effective learning relies on meaning rather than acquiring knowledge in a rote manner. Only by learning in context will the learner's previous knowledge be linked to new information. Experience lacking in reflection will remain unexamined and its potential for learning unrealized. Boychuk Duchscher (1999) identifies the active involvement in the process of your own practice in order to facilitate learning, whilst Eraut (1982) goes as far as to say that knowledge may have to be used before it can acquire any significant meaning for the user. Schön (1987) summed this up when he wrote:

> The paradox of learning a really new competence is this: that a student cannot at first understand what he needs to learn, can only learn it by educating himself through self discovery, and can only educate himself by beginning to do what he does not yet understand. (1987, p. 93)

This implies that you need to be involved in family care before you can understand what it is all about. Presentations of theoretical perspectives given before you have spent an adequate amount of time in practice are therefore not going to achieve any useful degree of understanding. It may even have deleterious effects. Overuse of terms such as 'family-centred care' or 'reflection' have been known to cause a certain 'groan' factor amongst students. Once the usefulness of reflection and family-centred care has been experienced, use of the expressions is more appropriate.

First discussions about family-centred care should therefore instil some key principles or rules that will ensure the student can begin to be involved and will be acting in an appropriate manner. It may be that such a strategy can be criticized for promoting an unthinking or routine approach to family-centred care; however, the real-life practice setting is an ill-structured and dynamic environment. Simple, memorable rules can provide a 'kick-start' for students to get involved, and they can also help students to make a positive contribution to the practice team. The importance of this is significant. 'Doing' is highly valued in the culture of nursing (Elzubeir and Sherman, 1995); student nurses naturally want to become valued and accepted members of the workforce (Mason and Jinks, 1994) and if students perceive that their skills are not developed sufficiently enough to be accepted as such, it can cause great anxiety (Neary, 1994).

So, what are these simple memorable rules and how can they help students begin to understand and experience family-centred care in the practice setting? For initial practice placements, student involvement should focus on simply *talking to the families.* Whilst this may be considered common sense and rather too obvious for words, an unfamiliar and sometimes frantically busy practice environment can make even the most confident new student feel at a loss for something to do. Often, students fill in time by reading notes or familiarizing themselves with equipment. Chatting to families can be seen as 'skiving'. Students may quickly find, however, that they learn just as much if not more from talking to families, than from any set of notes or piece of equipment. It may be useful for students to discuss with their mentors that they would like to spend some time talking to the families and perhaps identify it in their records as an objective to give themselves 'permission' to get involved in this activity.

Understandably, some students find it a little awkward at first, going up to families they have never met and striking up a conversation. Junior students can often shy away from interacting with families, maybe because of an inability to fall into easy conversation, or perhaps because of the perception that they need permission to do so. This may all sound a bit obvious, and those students who would naturally seek active interaction with families will do so anyway. Those who find it difficult, however, may benefit from discussing possible cues for conversation. For example:

● Ask if the child would like to play a game/read a book/watch a video, and use this to chat with the family about the child's likes and dislikes.

● Explain to the family that you are a junior student and you are looking for something to do to feel useful – is there anything you can do for them?

The other advantage of this type of involvement is that it can lead to the student being able to make a positive impact on the experience of children and families and provide very valuable feedback to the nursing team. Families will often talk to and ask questions of a learner or junior member of staff more readily than they might talk to a more senior nurse or doctor. This is partly circumstantial, – junior staff may spend more time in contact with the families and issues of concern to the family may then arise naturally in conversation. Also there is an element of safety for the family, in asking someone who is relatively low on the hierarchy of the practice setting. They may feel that the issues they are concerned about are perhaps too trivial to bother the busy nurses with, or they may be reluctant to make a fuss. Just listening and talking to families may be enough to improve their healthcare experience. Alternatively, the student's role may be feeding back to the rest of the nursing team any of the family's concerns or questions which he or she felt unable to deal with.

SCENARIO 7.1

Frances is 13 years old and is due to go to theatre today for a near total thyroidectomy. She is familiar enough with her condition and the operation itself to explain it all to Emma, a student nurse on the second week of her first-ever practice placement. Emma only met Frances and her mum, Margaret, today. The ward is fairly busy and Emma's mentor Jan is finding it difficult to go through things with Emma. She has asked Emma to spend some time talking to the families of the children in their care. Consequently, Emma has been spending time with Frances and Margaret while they have been waiting for the afternoon theatre list to get started.

While they are talking, Margaret asks how long Frances is likely to be away from the ward. Emma does not know. She has explained to Frances and Margaret that she is very new both to nursing and to the ward, and she suggests she goes to find out what she can from Jan. She comes back to say that Jan reckons Frances will be a while in the post-anaesthetic care unit but will be back probably by seven(ish) that evening. Frances quickly looks at her mum with a worried expression. Margaret holds her hand and tells Emma that Frances is prone to very heavy periods and that she started her period this morning. She is really worried that she will get in a bit of a mess in theatre or afterwards, before she comes back to the ward. Margaret said that she had mentioned this to a nurse earlier on, but nothing had been mentioned since. It was the one thing that Frances was most anxious about and she was too embarrassed to make a fuss about it. Emma said she would make sure Jan knew about this before Frances went to theatre. In fact, when Emma told her, Jan asked Emma to take a change of underwear and some of Frances' own sanitary towels to the post-anaesthetic care unit so that they could make sure her needs were adequately met. Both Margaret and Frances said that knowing this had been taken care of was enough to help them both cope much better with the day's events.

This scenario demonstrates how a junior member of the ward team with relatively little theoretical knowledge can still make a valuable contribution to the care of the family. The student may not have identified what she was doing using specific terminology, but she will be able use her experience and learn from it. The challenge is to find strategies that will evolve understanding and knowledge such that it can then be transferred back to the practice of the individual.

Beginning to reflect

Reflection and critical thinking have been proposed as tools to aid the integration of theory and practice in nursing (Boychuk Duchscher, 1999; Burns and Bulman, 1999; Palmer *et al.*, 1994). It is now more common than ever to see 'reflection' on student timetables. Reflection and critical thinking, however, are high-level cognitive skills, not easily developed even in optimum circumstances (Roberts *et al.*, 1992). In addition, much of effective nursing practice is implicit in its nature and is thus difficult to write down, let alone critique, even for experienced practitioners (Eraut, 1985).

Oakeshott (1962) used a distinction first described by Aristotle between 'technical knowledge' and 'practical knowledge'. Technical knowledge can be written down, but practical knowledge is expressed only in practice and learned only through practice. It is expecting a great deal of student nurses to both record and analyse their clinical experiences. Many students use their portfolios and learning diaries as somewhere to keep factual information about diseases, conditions and case histories, or to record events that occur in practice. Expecting more than this is to tread on uncertain ground. Eraut (1985) noted that self-knowledge of performance is difficult to acquire and self-comment tends to be justificatory rather than critical in intent. Written records can become more 'real' than actual events, the need to fill them in dominates and the type of knowledge demanded by the record determines what experience is sought.

The principles of reflection can be confusing and frustrating and students may feel that it has no relevance to them (Holm and Stephenson, 1994). Often this stage is a necessary precursor to understanding how the process works. Most students enter their training coming from a background of teacher-led activities in school. They do not know how to reflect on their experience and they are not sure if they want to. In order to get started it is necessary to know what questions to ask, what the teachers expect of students with regard to reflection, and where to start looking for the answers. Students need to get some experience in practice before they can be expected to begin learning about the process of reflection. They also need plenty of opportunities to practice reflective skills, which is why many courses now require reflective diaries or journals as part of the assessment of learning.

Entries in students' reflective diaries may initially be more descriptive than reflective, but their skills in this area will improve with practice. The important thing is to get into the habit of writing down things that are experienced in practice. This allows thoughts to be crystallized so that they can be examined. Overemphasis on the different reflective models and theories will be of limited value initially.

Practice staff can play an immensely important role in developing students' abilities to use reflection by helping them to identify the sorts of experiences that can be effectively utilized for the purpose. There may be some opportunities for student and mentor to reflect together on an experience, and this can be extremely useful for both. When this is not possible, mentors can advise students to write down a description of an experience, which they may be able to discuss together later, or for students to take back to the classroom setting. Choosing which incidents to record is actually very important. There is a tendency among students to record incidents which make reflection difficult or too complex to derive useful learning from at their stage of experience. The following is an example of a journal entry which a first year student, Katie, had chosen as a 'critical incident' for discussion:

> The ward was really busy and without warning through the doors came a trolley surrounded by doctors and nurses, with drips and machines and someone hand ventilating a child who we could barely make out beneath all the activity. The charge nurse was not expecting a patient let alone one who needed all this. It turned out the child was a boy with severe cerebral palsy who was very ill and was dying, but they didn't want him to die in the Accident and Emergency department so they brought him to our ward because they knew we had a cubicle free. The family were all with him and we had to find somewhere for them to wait while we sorted him out. It was mad and it took ages for everyone to settle down and get on with their work again. The boy actually survived for three whole days before he died. It was very stressful for everyone.

Students often believe 'critical' incidents to be emergencies, disasters and crises. The above incident is hugely complicated, and from the account it sounds as though Katie was more of an observer than an active participant. Now look at the following entry:

> Joe's mum was one of those people with stern faces. Some of the ward staff said she could be 'off' with them at times so I was a bit nervous when I was asked to look after Joe for the afternoon. Joe was lovely and we played a few games, but I was really scared that his mum might shout at me. She didn't laugh at my jokes or join in our game at all. She asked me about Joe's medicine. I didn't know and I really panicked. I thought, she's going to think she's got a right fool in charge of her son. I blurted out that I was only on my second ward placement and I hadn't met anyone with Joe's condition before and I was really sorry, but I could look it up or ask one of the other nurses. Then it was weird – she actually smiled.

Unlike the first extract, this journal entry would be better suited for early attempts at reflection because:

- it is personal;
- it is an experience in which Katie was an active participant; and
- it clearly left Katie in a state of confusion as to why things happened as they did.

In order to use this account, Katie can now be encouraged to ask herself some key questions to help her understand the experience:

- How did this incident make me feel?
- Why might Joe's mum have behaved the way she did?
- Why did her behaviour at first make me nervous, and then surprise me?
- Looking back on it, am I happy with way I behaved? Could I have handled it better?

The role of the facilitator here is to assist in the formulation of relevant questions or the use of appropriate reflective models. Early experiences of reflection need to be relevant, productive and interesting. Staff in the practice areas have an advantage here in that the relevance is obvious, and relevance is a key motivator. In school, teachers can use different strategies such as role play, simulation, clinical laboratory, use of scenarios from practice and so on to stimulate interest and debate. Some universities have utilized studios or arts laboratories with actors playing the parts of patients and their families, nursed by the students (Fitzgerald, 1994). Early benefit from these activities will help ensure students continue working at their reflective skills and participate in reflection so that it becomes an essential part of their practice.

The next steps: identifying the key concerns

SCENARIO 7.2

Shelley is 3 years old and has fallen off the climbing frame in her garden at home and bumped her head; she has a swelling on her forehead and is a little unsteady on her feet. She has also been sick once, shortly after arriving in the Accident and Emergency department. She has been admitted for observation, and arrived on the ward at 2.30 p.m. accompanied by her mother, Barbara. Shelley does not appear particularly unwell or unsteady, she has been playing with toys on her bed and has walked to the toilet unaided. Observation of Shelley so far has not given cause for concern. Barbara, however, seems edgy and anxious. She looks up nervously whenever a nurse or doctor walks into the room, and she has been trying to reach her husband on the ward payphone to organize someone to fetch her other two children, Jonathon (9 years) and Gavin (6 years) from school. When she did get through to him her voice had been raised and she was heard to shout angrily on a couple of occasions. She has also appeared to be getting impatient with Shelley who has responded by getting upset herself. When one of the nurses asked if everything was OK, Barbara snapped back with a sarcastic 'Oh yes, just great, couldn't be better', and then apologized briefly before returning to Shelley's bed.

What thoughts do you have reading through this scenario? How can you explain Barbara's behaviour? Here are some possibilities:

- She feels guilty because she was not watching Shelley on the climbing frame.
- She is worried about her other two children.
- She is worried that her husband will blame her for Shelley's accident.
- She is worried that Shelley is seriously injured.
- She may not have told the full story of the accident because it might incriminate her.

Any of these is possible and a nurse caring for Shelley and Barbara may well have thought of these possibilities. However, unless the nurse can quickly ascertain the true cause of Barbara's anxieties, the situation could deteriorate rapidly. This is because Barbara's anxious state is not due to any of the factors expressed above, but to an overwhelming fear of needles – she is needle phobic. The very sight of a needle could lead Barbara to have an anxiety attack or to faint but she is embarrassed to talk about it openly and feels that if she did she might be told that it would be better if she were to leave the ward. She does not want to risk having to leave Shelley on her own. Every time a doctor or nurse comes near, she panics thinking they may have a needle with them.

It is very easy to make assumptions based on our own experience and understanding. It is therefore important for students and their mentors to make explicit the notion of avoiding assumptions, particularly on initial assessment. The important point here is that Barbara's key concern is her fear of seeing a needle. It is not the most obvious or perhaps the most appropriate concern in the circumstances, but it is the one factor which is having the greatest impact on Barbara's experience and therefore will influence how well Shelley deals with her hospital stay.

A first stage in developing a useful and meaningful relationship with a family is therefore to establish exactly what are their key concerns. These may change over time, and different family members may be most concerned about different aspects of the situation, but if the nurse can deal with these adequately and appropriately, the relationship between nurse and family will be quickly established as a functional and beneficial one. Key concerns are often identified through an effective initial assessment interview and can be dealt with by appropriate planning of care. These early encounters with families are essential for the provision of effective care and therefore warrant a closer examination.

Planning care: an open and transparent process

SCENARIO 7.3

Janice, a 6-year-old with right orbital cellulitis, has been admitted for intravenous antibiotic therapy. Her dad, David, is present with her on admission to the ward. Apart from her swollen eye, Janice is not unwell. She had an intravenous cannula inserted in the Accident and Emergency department, and she and her dad have been shown to the bay which she will share with three other children, and she is sitting watching television when the nurse arrives to do her admission assessment. Janice has never been in hospital before and is quite excited at the thought of staying somewhere different. She has no brothers or sisters. Her mum works full-time as a financial advisor and David is a computer programmer working from home. He is Janice's main carer, confining his working hours to her school day, and he has said that he will be resident with Janice while she needs to be in hospital.

The nurse doing the admission assessment, Pippa, records a baseline temperature, pulse rate, respiratory rate, blood pressure, weight and height. She goes through Janice's normal routines for eating, drinking, playing, school work, sleep, and going to the toilet. Pippa asks about medications, allergies, whether Janice's sight and hearing are OK and any particular toys or special words she might have which the nursing staff ought to be made aware of. Pippa takes David and Janice on a tour of the ward, pointing out the patient toilet, the parent toilet, the play room and the sitting room. Pippa tells David where the dining room is and what time meals are served. She also tells him what sleeping arrangements he can expect. Pippa finishes the admission by saying that if he has any questions, he only has to ask. David did not have any particular questions and since he saw very little of Pippa for the rest of the day, he did not speak with her again.

Is there anything wrong with this? Perhaps nothing drastic, but Pippa is keeping the process very much under her own control. Now consider an alternative scenario:

SCENARIO 7.4

When Pippa introduced herself to David and Janice she explained that she wanted to put together a plan for looking after Janice 'so we all know what we should be doing'. Pippa briefly went through what Janice and David could expect during their stay in hospital, including how often she would need her medicine, how it would be given, and for how many days. Pippa gave reasons for everything she did, from taking Janice's temperature to going through her home routines. Janice and David were shown the documentation Pippa was using, and she then went on to ask about how Janice and David would like the nursing staff to be involved in Janice's care. Pippa explained that, generally, parents liked to remain responsible for things like comforting, washing and dressing, feeding and playing. Once they had discussed what Janice and David thought would be appropriate, Pippa wrote it in the documentation and showed them what she had written. Pippa then went on to suggest they did the same for aspects of care such as giving oral medications and taking Janice's temperature. Pippa pointed out that for Janice's condition, where her need for hospitalization was likely to be fairly brief and not repeated, it was perhaps unrealistic to talk about David getting involved with her intravenous antibiotics, but if he wanted to know more about this she would certainly discuss it with him.

Once Pippa, David and Janice had come up with a plan of care, Pippa told them that they could see how it goes and, if necessary, change it to fit their needs. David was keen that Janice's mum could see and possibly change the plan when she arrived after she had finished work. Pippa suggested that David show his wife the plan when she arrived so that they could discuss it. Once they had done this, Pippa said she would come and go through anything they were concerned about. They agreed this plan and then Pippa showed Janice and David around the ward.

Janice did not require her next antibiotics until later on that evening, but Pippa frequently came by for a quick chat or to ask if they needed anything.

Some key points in comparing scenario 7.4 with scenario 7.3 are as follows:

- Both admissions would have taken about the same length of time; busyness does not prevent an alternative approach being taken.
- In the second admission scenario, Janice and her father could see and influence what was being written about them.
- In the second scenario, Janice and her dad were aware of what they could expect and what was expected of them. They also knew how to change the arrangement and had frequent access to Pippa in order to do so.

It is quite possible, even likely, that there would be very little observable difference between family participation after the first admission process and family participation after the second admission process. The way David and Janice *felt* about their experience, however, is likely to be quite different. This demonstrates the distinction between parent participation and family-centred care. The key factors for the admission process are therefore:

- explain why you are asking the questions;
- suggest it is up to the family to be the major influence on what aspects of care will be your responsibility, rather than the other way around; and
- share with the family what you are writing down, and actually show them the documentation.

Be visible

Once the admission assessment is complete, one other fundamental rule must be brought into play: make sure you frequently 'check in' on the family, even if there is not a lot to do for them. Long periods with no interest shown in you can be boring, frustrating, worrying or even maddening. It is easily dealt with and can avoid upset and confrontation.

Summary

So, in summary, a step-by-step guide for students new to family-centred care would be as follows:

- talk to patients;
- start to record interesting experiences;
- acknowledge the tendency to make assumptions about people and avoid this;
- try to identify the family's key concerns and deal with them appropriately;
- make the planning of care as transparent as possible;
- explain why you need specific information;
- show the child and family the documentation you are using for their admission assessment;
- agree a process for reviewing your plan of care; and
- maintain a presence – be seen often.

These are perhaps oversimplified, but whilst the more complex nature of family-centred care is a highly significant area of development for children's nurses, major concerns exist about the basic aspects being effectively implemented in practice. Early experiences in the practice setting can be confusing and scary, particularly when combined with expectations of academic assignments that need to be done, and journals or diaries that need to be filled with something appropriate. This chapter has attempted to untangle some of these issues in order to support students as they begin to practice family-centred care. The range of legal and professional issues raised by sharing care with families will be explored next in Chapter 8.

References

Ausubel, D. P., Novak, J. D. and Hanesian, H. (1978) *Educational Psychology, a Cognitive View*, 2nd edn (New York: Holt, Rinehart & Winston).

Boychuk Duchscher, J. E. (1999) 'Catching the Wave: Understanding the Concept of Critical Thinking', *Journal of Advanced Nursing*, 29(3), pp. 577–83

Burns, S. and Bulman, C. (1999) *Reflective Practice in Nursing: The Growth of the Professional Practitioner* (Blackwell Science).

Elzubeir, M. and Sherman, M. (1995) 'Nursing Skills and Practice', *British Journal of Nursing*, 4(18), pp. 1087–92.

Eraut, M. (1982) 'What is Learned in In-service Education and How? A Knowledge User Perspective', *British Journal of In-Service Training*, 9(1), pp. 6–14.

Eraut, M. (1985) *Knowledge Creation and Use in Professional Contexts. Studies in Higher Education*, 10(2), pp. 117–33.

Eraut, M., Alderton, J., Boylon, A. and Wright, A. (1995) *Confusions and Clarifications about Theory and Practice*, ENB Research Report No 3, pp. 9–10.

Fitzgerald, M. (1994) 'Theories of Reflection for Learning', in A. Palmer, S. Burns and C. Bulman (eds), *Reflective Practice in Nursing: The Growth of the Professional Practitioner* (London: Blackwell), chapter 5, pp. 63–84.

French, P. (1992) 'The Quality of Nurse Education in the 1980s', *Journal of Advanced Nursing*, 17, pp. 619–31.

Gray, M. and Smith, L. N. (1999) 'The Professional Socialization of Diploma of Higher Education in Nursing Students: A Longitudinal Study', *Journal of Advanced Nursing*, 29(3), pp. 639–47.

Greenwood, J. (1993) 'The Apparent Desensitization of Student Nurses During their Professional Socialisation: A Cognitive Perspective', *Journal of Advanced Nursing*, 18, pp. 1471–9.

Holm, D. and Stephenson, S. (1994) 'Reflection – A Student's Perspective', in A. Palmer, S. Burns and C. Bulman (eds), *Reflective Practice in Nursing: The Growth of the Professional Practitioner* (London: Blackwell), chapter 4, pp. 53–62.

Hislop, S., Inglis, B., Cope, P., Stoddart, B. and McIntosh, C. (1996) 'Situating Theory in Practice: Students' Views of Theory–Practice in Project 2000 Nursing Programmes', *Journal of Advanced Nursing*, 23, pp. 171–7.

Johns, C. (2000) *Becoming a Reflective Practitioner* (Blackwell Science).

Mason, G. and Jinks, A. (1994) 'Examining the Role of the Practitioner-Teacher in Nursing', *British Journal of Nursing*, 3(20), pp. 1063–72.

Neary, M. (1994) 'Teaching Practical Skills in Colleges', *Nursing Standard*, 30 March, 8(27), pp. 35–8.

Oakeshott, M. (1962) *Rationalism in Politics: and Other Essays* (London: Heinemann).

Palmer, A., Burns, S. and Bulman, C. (eds) (1994) *Reflective Practice in Nursing: The Growth of the Professional Practitioner* (London: Blackwell).

Pounds, L. A. (1989) 'Beyond Florence Nightingale: The General Professional Education of the Nurse', *Academic Medicine*, 64(2), pp. 67–9.

Procter, S. (1989) 'The Functioning of Nursing Routines in the Management of a Transient Workforce', *Journal of Advanced Nursing*, 14, pp. 180–9.

Roberts, J., While, A. E. and Fitzpatrick, J. M. (1992) 'Simulation: Current Status in Nurse Education', *Nurse Education Today*, 12, pp. 409–15.

Schön, D. (1987). *Educating the Reflective Practitioner: Toward a New Design for Teaching and Learning in the Professions* (San Francisco: Jossey-Bass).

United Kingdom Central Council for Nursing Midwifery and Health Visiting (1999) *Fitness for Practice* (London: UKCC).

8

Professional and Legal Issues

Lynne Foxcroft*

Introduction

Family-centred care is an innovative approach to caring for children and young people in hospital and at home, which entails the delegation by nurses and other healthcare professionals to the parents of some general caring and nursing procedures. This delegation of care reduces the level of direct control, which the nurse has traditionally exercised over the charges in his/her care, and this could create an environment in which things may go wrong, and so increase the possibility of allegations of negligence against the nurses. Therefore family-centred care creates for the healthcare professional a range of professional and legal issues which need to be addressed and resolved in order that s/he may confidently participate in the scheme. The purpose of this chapter is to describe to the reader and alert him/her to the basis of potential legal and professional liability which is relevant to family-centred care. The chapter will also suggest measures which, if introduced, could assist the practitioner in avoiding the potential professional and legal pitfalls. The bases of liability to be considered are negligence, professional misconduct and occupier's liability.

* The author would like to express a debt of gratitude to Melanie Fellowes, a colleague, and the staff of the Children's Services Department of the Leeds General Infirmary for their time and invaluable assistance in the writing of this chapter.

Negligence

The incidence of negligence actions against healthcare professionals has increased dramatically over the last two decades. This increase has probably been fostered by an increased awareness by the general public of the access to law and the current compensation culture. If a negligence action is successful, not only will damages be payable but it could have a profound effect on a practitioner's career. Therefore it is essential that every practitioner should be aware of what must be proved for a negligence action to be successful, and to recognize the risks in his/her daily work so as to avoid liability.

The principles of negligence and family-centred care

Negligence is a tort, or civil wrong, which has been described as the

> omission to do something which a reasonable man guided by those considerations which ordinarily regulate the conduct of human affairs would do or doing something which a prudent and reasonable man would not do. (*Blyth* v. *Birmingham Waterworks Co.* (1856) 11 Exch 781)

For a negligence action to be successful, the plaintiff (the person claiming in negligence) must prove three things against the defendant (the person against whom the claim is made):

- that the defendant owed the plaintiff a duty of care;
- that the defendant breached his duty of care; and
- that damage/injury was caused by the breach.

To be successful, *all three* elements must be proved on the balance of probabilities (whether it is more likely than not that the defendant was negligent). If the plaintiff is unable to prove one of more of these three elements, then negligence cannot be established. These three elements are now considered with particular reference to family-centred care.

Duty of care

By whom is the duty owed?

The defendant must prove that s/he was owed a duty of care. This duty may be owed by the nurse and/or the NHS Trust.

- *The nurse*   A nurse or other healthcare professional may owe a duty of care. Establishing a duty of care is not usually a problem, since by admitting a child into hospital and providing care for him/her, a duty has either expressly or impliedly arisen.
- *The NHS Trust*   If there is an allegation of negligence against a nurse, the National Health Service Trust, as the nurse's employer, could also be found liable for his/her alleged negligence on a number of grounds. Firstly, the Trust's liability could arise on the basis of vicarious liability – an employment-law principle which establishes that an employer is liable for the torts (or civil wrongs, of which negligence is one) of his employees which are committed in the course of their employment. The Trust is still liable even though the nurse performs his/her duties negligently (*Iqbal* v. *London Transport Executive* (1973) 16 KIR 329), for example if the nurse were to give medication to the wrong patient. The Trust is vicariously liable even if the nurse did something which she had been specifically prohibited to do (*Rose* v. *Plenty* [1976] 1 WLR 141), for example if a junior nurse ignored an instruction that she should never allow a parent to administer injections. However, the employer will *not* be liable if the nurse goes beyond the scope of his/her employment duties (*Century Insurance Co.* v. *Northern Ireland Road Transport Board* [1942] AC 509), for example if s/he should smack a child.

    The Trust may not be vicariously liable for the negligence of agency nurses who work within the Trust's hospitals since they are probably regarded as employees of the agency. The relationship of the agency to the Trust is that of an independent contractor, and employment law has established that employers (the Trust) are not vicariously liable for the torts of their independent contractors. The Trust could only be liable for the negligence of an agency nurse if the Trust had been in breach of its duty to provide its patients with reasonable care by using the services of a sub-standard agency.

Secondly, since 1990, under the principle of Crown indemnity NHS Trusts are required to assume all responsibility for the negligence of their employees when the negligence is caused during the course of employment.

Thirdly, it has been established that a Trust owes a direct duty of care towards its patients. This includes a duty to employ suitably qualified and competent staff and to ensure that they are adequately supervised, so as to provide patients with a reasonably safe and effective standard of care (*Bull* v. *Devon Area Health Authority* (1993) 4 Ned LR 117).

Therefore a negligence claim may be made against a nurse or his/her employer. However, it is likely that the action will be brought against the employer since the Trust is better placed to provide adequate compensation.

To whom is the duty owed?

To recognise potential liability for negligence, the nurse must be aware of the extent of his/her duty of care – to whom is this duty owed? In *Donoghue* v. *Stevenson* [1932] AC 562, the House of Lords (the Court of the highest authority in England) established that a duty of care is owed to those who may foreseeably be harmed by one's actions (the neighbour principle):

> you must take reasonable care to avoid acts or omissions which you can reasonably foresee would be likely to injure your neighbour. Who, then, is my neighbour? The answer seems to be persons who are so closely and directly affected by my acts that I ought to have them in contemplation as being so affected when I am directing my mind to the acts or omissions that are called in question.

Therefore, the nurse on the ward will have a *specific* duty to his/her child patient. In family-centred care the nurse will also owe a duty to the parents, for example to provide adequate information and supervision. For example, if a nurse were to give incorrect instructions to a parent concerning the administration of insulin injections to a child, as a result of which the child suffered injury and the parent suffered psychological harm. The nurse would owe a duty of care and be liable to both parties, since it is forseeable that they would both be affected by his/her acts and that because of these acts foresight of damage is reasonable. It could therefore be established that the nurse owed a duty of care to both parents and child.

In addition s/he will owe a *general* duty of care to anyone who may foreseeably be harmed by any negligent acts or omissions. For example if a child patient's sibling suffered psychological harm after witnessing the effects on the patient of a nurse's negligence, then the nurse would be liable because it is foreseeable that a sibling will visit the patient and become distressed by witnessing the harm caused.

Breach of duty

It has been established that the healthcare professional owes a duty of care, but for a negligence action to be successful it must be also be proved that this duty was breached – that the healthcare professional's conduct was below the standard which is required and expected. Therefore s/he must be aware of the required standard of care.

The duty of care: the standard?

The general law of negligence requires that the defendant's acts should be measured against the standard of the reasonable (or the average) person (*Blyth* v. *Birmingham Waterworks Co.* (1856) 11 Exch 781). This is an objective test – how would the reasonable person have acted, and did the defendant act as the reasonable person would have acted? However, this standard is inappropriate within a professional medical context which requires skills which the reasonable person does not possess, and so a further test has been devised (the Bolam test):

> The test is the standard of the ordinary skilled man exercising and professing to have that special skill ... a failure to act in accordance with the standards of reasonably competent

medical men at the time. (*Bolam* v. *Friern Hospital Management Committee* [1957] 1 WLR 582)

Therefore as long as the nurse 'acts in accordance with a practice accepted at the time as proper by a responsible body of nursing opinion', s/he will not have breached his/her duty of care. Appropriate standards are those which are accepted within the profession and specifically those established by the UKCC (2000). If there are two reasonably competent bodies of opinion on an issue, a nurse will not be negligent if she follows one or other. However, it was held by the House of Lords in *Bolitho* v. *City and Hackney Health Authority* (No2) [1997] 4 All ER 771, that even though a practitioner may act in accordance with a responsible body of opinion, s/he may still be negligent if this practice does not stand up to logical analysis. The courts have thus reserved the right to act as the final arbiter when deciding the standard of care in medical negligence. An error of judgment does not in itself create liability if it follows professional practice and is reasonably well-informed.

For example if a nurse acts in compliance with accepted nursing practice but in *those* particular circumstances that action is inappropriate or unwise, s/he may nevertheless be found liable in negligence by the court. The House of Lords held that this principle established in *Bolitho* should apply to diagnosis and treatment, but did not specifically refer to its application to the disclosure of risks to patients. The nurse would avoid liability if s/he followed accepted professional practice when disclosing any risks, thus satisfying the Bolam test. The Bolam test has been widely criticized because it effectively leaves the standard of care to be decided solely by the medical profession, and is considered by some to be heavily weighted against the plaintiff. However, the current emphasis on clinical governance and the following of nationwide standards and procedures should mean that the question of breach of duty might eventually be taken away from the professions and addressed more objectively.

Negligence actions may take years to reach the courts, but a nurse will be judged against the standards which were in keeping at the time of the incident in which the alleged negligence arose. In *Roe* v. *Ministry of Health* [1954] 2 QB 66, the plaintiff was paralysed by an anaesthetic which had been contaminated by phenol which had seeped through invisible cracks in the glass phials in which the anaesthetic was stored. This risk was unknown at the time of the incident and so the defendant was held not to be negligent – the defendant had not fallen below the standards expected of him *at that time.*

The duty of care: the inexperienced nurse

It has been established above that a nurse must act in accordance with accepted professional practice, and a strict application of this principle means that the same standard of skill would be required of a newly-qualified nurse as that required of an experienced nurse. The standard is that of the ordinary competent practitioner – inexperience is no defence (*Nettleship* v. *Weston* [1971] 3 All ER 581). However, the courts have recognized that the present healthcare system requires that practitioners are expected to learn on the job and that their inexperience makes them vulnerable. Therefore the House of Lords in *Wilsher* v. *Essex Area Health Authority* [1987] QB 730 related the standard of the duty of care to the post which the practitioner occupies. They established that the standard of care expected is that of the averagely competent and well-informed practitioner in *that* particular position. For example, in *Wilsher* an inexperienced doctor mistakenly placed a catheter to monitor the oxygen level of a premature baby's blood into a vein instead of into an artery. As a result, excessive oxygen was administered which allegedly caused the child's sight to suffer. A more senior doctor, who failed to notice the mistake, checked the junior doctor's work. It was held that the senior doctor was negligent but that his junior colleague was not – he had acted reasonably in his junior post by acknowledging his inexperience and having his work checked. Therefore an inexperienced nurse must act reasonably within the post she occupies. For example, if she were asked by a parent for some advice which she did not feel competent to give, she would discharge her duty by recognizing her inexperience and ask a senior nurse for assistance. If she did not do so, she would be negligent since she would not have acted as would a reasonably competent nurse with the same level of experience. It follows that nurse managers and ward sisters in turn owe a duty to their patients to ensure that inexperienced nurses are adequately supervised and monitored.

The duty of care and family-centred care

It has been established above that negligence may be committed by both acts and omissions, so the nurse may be liable if s/he both negligently gives a parent incorrect advice or if s/he negligently omits to advise the parents. It has also been established that when discharging his/her duty to patients, the nurse owes a duty to act in accordance with a body of responsible medical opinion and in doing so should follow approved professional nursing practice (UKCC, 1992). General standards of approved practice have not been established for family-centred care and so consideration will now be given to specific aspects of the procedure.

Recruiting the participants in family-centred care
Both parents and the child may participate in family-centred care and so to discharge his/her duty of care the nurse must be aware of the following issues:

- *For parents*   When recruiting potential parents to participate in family-centred care, the nurse owes a duty to his/her patients to ensure that those parents who participate will have the ability to perform the necessary functions, the capacity to be responsive to the instructions they are given, and will act reliably and responsibly. S/he should therefore be aware of any possibility of child abuse or of Munchausen's Syndrome by Proxy. Although the nurse will have to use his/her professional judgment to decide whether or not a parent has the capacity to participate in the child's care, it is also important that a parent is not prejudged, and that each parent is given the opportunity to learn a procedure, even if that means extending the training process. This would fulfil the nurse's duty to both child patient and parent, recognizing that parental involvement is in most cases beneficial to both parties.
  The practice on the ward may be to allow parents to give as much assistance as they feel capable of in the general care of the child. A care plan should generally be negotiated with the family so that all concerned are certain as to each person's role in the care of the child and the procedures which will be

taken during the child's stay in hospital. The care plan should be documented once both staff and parent understand the agreed plan.

The Hospital Trust would have a duty to provide relevant training of staff with regard to the assessment of parents' abilities in order to meet its own duty of care to the patient.

- *For children*   Current paediatric nursing practice establishes that hospitalization may entail a loss of independence for the young person, and that the young person should be encouraged to participate in decision-making and treatment and, if possible, that their opinions and wishes should be respected (Smith, 1995). It is important to establish that the nurse owes a duty to ensure that the initiation of any delegation is in accordance with acceptable professional practice. To enable him/her to discharge that duty it is vital to identify when a young person may make valid healthcare decisions and participate in patient care.

  It is accepted that a young person between the age of 16 and 18 years is capable of giving valid consent to surgical and medical treatment (Section 8(1) Family Law Reform Act 1969), but his/her *refusal* of treatment may be overridden by the courts or by those with parental responsibility (*Re W (A Minor)(Medical Treatment: Court's Jurisdiction)* [1993] Fam 64). The legality of consent of a young person under the age of 16 is more problematic. Those who have parental responsibility for the young person may give consent to treatment for him/her, but the young person may have the capacity to give consent on their own behalf. The test of capacity is not based on chronological age, but on whether the young person has achieved a sufficient degree of maturity and intelligence to enable them to understand the nature and implications of the proposed treatment (Gillick competency – established by the House of Lords in *Gillick* v. *West Norfolk and Wisbech Area Health Authority* [1986] 1 AC 112.

  It will be a matter of professional judgment for the nurse to decide whether the young person has sufficient understanding and intelligence. The nurse should take into account the nature of the proposed treatment and the young person's ability to fully understand and appraise the risk, and the implications and consequences of receiving the treatment or not receiving the treatment. The Gillick test of competency is limited on two grounds. Firstly it is only applicable to consent to treatment (a parent or the court may override a young person's refusal of treatment), and secondly it only applies to the staged development of a normal child, not, for example, in a situation in which the child suffers from fluctuating mental disability (*In re R (A Minor)(Wardship: Consent to Treatment)* [1992] Fam 11). The degree of understanding required of the child will be commensurate with the seriousness and degree of complexity of the proposed treatment, since the young person must understand and appreciate the consequences of treatment, non-treatment and the possible side-effects. There is a difference, for example, between the understanding required to record one's fluid balance and that required to administer one's insulin injections.

Delegation and supervision

Family-centred care involves both the delegation of some nursing procedures to others and the consequent supervision of that care.

● *Delegation* When deciding to delegate, the nurse has a duty to ensure that the child is treated appropriately and that adequate care is provided so that the child does not suffer harm. Therefore the nurse has a duty to take reasonable care and to follow approved practice. Dimond (1990) identifies that to discharge this duty the nurse should ensure that:

○ *It is appropriate to delegate that task to that specific parent.* The nurse should not delegate until she feels entirely secure in the knowledge that the parent is able to undertake the relevant care. Some parents may consider that they are capable of taking on certain areas of care yet the nurse may not feel as secure. Should the nurse be intimidated into handing over care, then she may not be fulfilling his/her duty of care to the child. Children should not be placed in a position where their health is jeopardized. For this reason nurses will themselves require training in order to assess parents' competency, and how to negotiate with them as to what aspects of the child's care they are able to assume. This should not be an extra burden which is placed on the nurse without support or training as this in itself could lead to a breach of a primary duty of the hospital, that is a duty to provide a safe system of work.

○ *The parent has been given enough information to ensure that the task can be carried out reasonably safely.* Therefore the nurse owes a duty of care to the child, his/her patient, to the parent who should be adequately instructed and supervised, and to anyone else whose harm may be reasonably foreseeable.

● *Supervision* By instigating family-centred care the nurse has created a duty to supervise that care. To discharge that duty the nurse should provide supervision of the parent, which is adequate to ensure that the parent is sufficiently competent to undertake the treatment before being allowed to act alone. To discharge his/her duty to the patient, the nurse will be required to assess the competence and experience of the parent. The assessment should be based on the nurse's clinical judgment of the parent's skill and competence, which should also be subject to the standards of appropriate professional practice. The factors upon which the assessment should be made include:

(i)   *The nature of the task.* The demands on the parent can vary from having to perform a relatively simple task such as assisting with toileting, to changing a stoma dressing, to carrying out traction or learning how to put a nappy on a child with hip spica.

(ii)   *The qualifications and experience of the parent.* Although these factors may influence the nurse's decision it is also important not to presume too quickly that a parent will be unable to carry out certain tasks without allowing him/her the opportunity to learn how to perform a procedure.

(iii) *Any reasonably foreseeable risks.* Given the nurse's professional status it would be for the nurse to foresee any possible risks attached to the parent being delegated a certain task. For example, if a parent is assessed as able to administer medication there is a foreseeable risk that the medication could be duplicated – administered by the parent *and* by a member of staff, thus endangering the patient.

The NHS Trust has a primary duty to provide a safe system of work for its employees and in order to discharge that duty should ensure that the nursing staff receive adequate support and training.

Instruction
Dimond (1990) suggests that in order to discharge his/her duty of care the nurse should take reasonable care to ensure that any instructions given are:

- *Comprehensive.* For example, if a parent is told that he or she can give a child a drink before an operation as the child is becoming dehydrated, then it must be made clear what type and quantity of fluid is appropriate and how near the expected time of operation it can safely be given.
- *Communicated appropriately.* Verbal communication of instructions may be insufficient and it may be more prudent to provide written instructions. These will give the parent something to refer to if in doubt and will avoid the situation where the instructions were given at a time of stress for both parents and staff. It is important that appropriate language and terminology are used to ensure that the parents understand them and feel confident about the relevant procedures.
- *Sufficiently adequate to ensure that the recipient is safe.* The wellbeing of the child must be the prime motivation for everyone involved in his/her care and the practitioner has a duty to ensure that the information and instruction are provided within this context. It must be recognized by the nursing staff that parents may be unfamiliar with certain terms and may not always see risks which are obvious to the experienced professional. It should also be made clear to the parent that they should do no more than they have been trained or instructed to do, and to assist all parties instructions should preferably be in writing. This will provide evidence that the nurse's duty to both patient and parent has been carried out and will also help the parent as he or she will have something to refer to.

Some large NHS Trusts have appointed specialist nurses who are not ward-based and whose duties are hospital-wide and who instruct parents in the care of their child, for example diabetes nurses.

It should also be made clear to parents that the training given is relevant only to their own child and that no action should be taken on behalf of another child without a member of staff being asked. The parent may have the very best of intentions yet could inadvertently harm another child, not being fully informed of the case history of that particular patient.

The nurse also has a general duty to ensure that all parents are aware of safety procedures in respect of their own and others' children. The issues include, *inter alia* that the kitchen door should always be kept closed, that hot drinks should not be taken on to the ward, and that extreme care should be taken in respect of harmful substances. It will be a matter of professional judgment as to the manner in which the instructions are given and the pace of the learning process. If the nurse negligently instructs his/her parents, or does so in such a way that they do not understand the instructions, and the patient is harmed, the nurse could be in breach of duty and liable in negligence for that harm.

Disclosure of risks
When disclosing any possible risks of treatment to the patient the nurse should conform to the standard established by the Bolam test – that s/he should follow the accepted practice of a responsible body of medical opinion (*Sidaway* v. *Bethlem Royal Hospital* [1985] AC 871). The nurse is under a duty to disclose material risks, those which a reasonable person in the parents' position would regard as significant to know. Exceptionally, the nurse may exercise his/her clinical judgment and so be justified in not disclosing a risk if that information would adversely affect the child's health or well-being.

Duty to keep up to date
The nurse has a duty to keep up to date with developments in nursing care generally (including family-centred care) but s/he does not have a duty to read every article appearing in the nursing/medical press (*Crawford* v. *Charing Cross Hospital* (1953)

Times, 8 Dec.). However, there is a duty to keep generally informed on mainstream changes in practice through the major journals and textbooks (*Gascoigne* v. *Ian Sheridan & Co.* [1994] 5 Med LR 437).

The duty of care in specific tasks within a hospital environment

(i)   *Feeding.* Feeding is generally included in the day-to-day care of the child and it is probably one of the first tasks that a parent will wish to assume. To discharge their duty of care, nurses should ensure that they have given parents very clear and specific instructions as to when and how children should be fed and what type of food may be given. Even the simple task of providing food can have disastrous consequences if the parent is misinformed or ignorant of certain facts, for example if the patient is about to undergo surgery the parents should clearly understand what food/drink is permissible and when these should be discontinued.

(ii) *Toileting.* The nurse has a duty to inform the parents of any procedures or restrictions concerning the child's toileting. For example, whether the child is allowed to get out of bed to go to the toilet, what the parents should be looking for, what to do if the child is clearly showing pain, how often the child is needing to go to the toilet, and whether or not the child should be allowed to go, for example a full bladder may be required for an ultrasound scan.

(iii) *Administering medicines.* The administration of medicines may be delegated to parents. In some family-centred care schemes drugs are stored in a lockable cabinet by the child's bed and the parents are responsible for the administration and recording of the medication. The nurse will have a duty to ensure that the parents are adequately instructed and supervised in this procedure. The NHS Trust would have a corresponding duty to ensure that nurses received adequate supervision and that appropriate procedures have been established. The UKCC have acknowledged that the administration of medicines may be delegated to informal carers who might be instructed accordingly, and that the decision to delegate may be left to the professional judgement of the practitioner (UKCC, 2000).

The duty of care in the home environment
It is now well-established that a child will generally be happier and so more likely to improve if in his/her home environment. If the child requires continued medical care whilst at home, the NHS Trust has a duty to ensure that the parents will have received adequate instruction before the child is discharged and that they receive supervision and back-up facilities after discharge. The nurses have a duty to ensure that the parents are willing and able to undertake the responsibility of continuing care at home and that they receive suitable training. After discharge, the child will be in the care of the community care providers who will then be responsible for his/her healthcare. The need for adequate communication, support, documentation and instruction is particularly important in the home environment.

If the community nurse is negligent then his/her employer (possibly the Primary Care Group) will be vicariously liable. A patient's General Practitioner may be liable as an employer, but the NHS Trust will not be liable for a GP's negligence, since a GP has the status of an independent contractor.

Damage was caused by the negligence

If the plaintiff has proved that the defendant owed him a duty of care and that the duty was breached, s/he must still prove that the breach of duty caused the harm in respect of which the claim is made. Relevant damage may include damage or loss to property, illness, physical injury, the exacerbation of an existing condition, psychiatric injury, pain and suffering and possibly financial loss.

Establishing causation

Establishing causation is often difficult within a medical setting for a number of reasons. Firstly, a patient may be suffering from a number of conditions which could have caused the harm, and the courts have often taken a favourable stance in respect of healthcare professionals and causation (*R* v. *Cheshire* [1991] 3 All ER 670). Secondly, it must be proved on the balance of probabilities (more likely than not) that the breach caused the harm, not merely that this/here was a chance that it might have done so.

A basic factual test to establish causation is the 'but for' test, which asks the question, 'but for the defendant's actions would the plaintiff have suffered the injury?' If the answer is 'no', liability could be established, if the answer is 'yes' then the injury would have occurred regardless and no liability arises. For example, in *Barnet* v. *Chelsea and Kensington HMC* [1969] 1 QB 428, a negligence action against a doctor failed because, although the doctor had breached his duty by turning a patient away from casualty without being examined, the doctor had not caused the patient's death. The death was caused by arsenic poisoning which would have been untreatable even if the patient had been examined.

The 'but for' test is a good factual starting point in establishing causation but it is not totally determinative because there may be more than one possible cause of the harm. The legal cause of the injury must therefore be established, and this may be done by asking whether the defendant's negligent act has materially contributed to the injury (*Bonnington Castings Ltd* v. *Wardlaw* [1956] AC 613). For example, a nurse may administer a drug to a patient in a dosage which, although in excess of the prescribed dose, is not lethal, and the patient who has a hitherto undiscovered sensitivity to the drug suffers an allergic reaction and dies. An application of the 'but for' test establishes that but for the nurse's actions the patient would not have died, but that the real cause of death was his abnormal sensitivity to the drug.

Negligence may be committed not only by an act but also by an omission, which could cause the patient's condition to deteriorate. In *Bolitho* a hospital doctor did not attend a child with breathing difficulties and therefore did not intubate. The House of Lords held that it had to be established, firstly, whether the doctor would have intubated if she had attended, and secondly, if she would not have done so, whether a reasonably competent practitioner would also not have intubated. Therefore the effect of *Bolitho* is that it applies the Bolam test into causation – when omission by causation is in issue, a practitioner may be judged against the standard of a reasonably competent body of opinion.

The chain of causation

If a nurse is to be liable for an injury caused by his/her negligence there must be a 'chain of causation', which links the injury with the negligence. If this chain of causation is broken the nurse is not liable. The chain may be broken by an act which intervenes between the defendant's negligence and the injury, and which is so unconnected as to be regarded as the new cause of the injury. An example of an intervening act could be the acts of third parties. For example, if a friend of the parent in a family-centred care scheme were to attempt the child's care in the parent's absence and the child suffered injury as a result, this could break the chain of causation. However, the nurse could still be in breach of his/her duty if s/he had omitted to instruct the parents that they must not delegate their care to another or allow another to treat the child.

Res ipsa loquitur – an exception to the burden of proof

In negligence the plaintiff must prove that the defendant was negligent. However *res ipsa loquitur* (the thing speaks for itself) is an exception to this rule – by which the courts will infer that the defendant has been negligent and therefore s/he must show that the injury could have resulted without negligence on his/her part. *Res ipsa loquitur* is rarely invoked, and will be relevant when the only explanation for the injury in question is that the defendant has been negligent, for example if a swab is left inside a patient after an operation. For *res ipsa loquitur* to be successful it must be established that the defendant has 'control' of the thing or circumstance which caused the damage, and that the accident is one which does not happen in the ordinary course of events in the absence of negligence (*Barkway* v. *South Wales Transport Company Ltd* [1950] AC 185).

Remoteness of damage

Even though the defendant has been negligent and the negligence has caused the harm, s/he may not be liable for the all the harm caused if it is established that this harm is too far removed from the injury – if it is too remote. The test as to whether the harm is too remote from the practitioner's negligence is whether the harm is a reasonably foreseeable consequence of the defendant's breach of duty (*The Wagon Mound* [1962] AC 388). Therefore the harm may not be reasonably foreseeable if it is of a different type than that expected or if it occurred in a different way from that which was expected. For example, a nurse will be liable if s/he negligently instructs the mother as to the care of the child patient and, as a result, the child suffers reasonably foreseeable physical injury. The nurse would be liable both for the child's injuries and any psychiatric condition which was suffered by the mother as a result of inadvertently harming his/her own child. However, she may not be liable for the losses incurred by the child's father who temporarily abandons his business interests to be with his child – these are not reasonably foreseeable and therefore too remote.

Liability for a nurse's negligence, which causes nervous shock to a person who witnesses the aftermath of a negligent incident arises when the following criteria are satisfied:

- The nurse's conduct must have resulted in a medically recognizable illness or condition caused by a sudden/immediate shock (not just feelings of fear or distress). For example, if parents suffer clinical depression or post-traumatic stress disorder as a result of the death or injury to their child which has been caused by the nurse's negligence (*Tredget and Tredget* v. *Bexley Health Authority* [1994] 5 Med LR 178).
- It was reasonably foreseeable that a reasonably brave person would have reacted in the way that the plaintiff did (thereby excluding the over-sensitive parent).
- The plaintiff was sufficiently proximate (or near to) the accident; here there are two aspects:

(i) The plaintiff must have been present personally or witnessed the tragedy or its immediate aftermath – not through a third party.

(ii) It must be proved that the plaintiff had a close bond of love and affection with the victim (*Alcock* v. *Chief Constable of South Yorkshire* [1991] 4 All ER 907). This will not present a problem if the plaintiff is the child's parent.

An exception to the rule on remoteness of damage – the 'thin skull' rule – may extend the practitioner's liability. This rule establishes that the defendant must take his victim as he finds him in mind as well as in body – if s/he has a latent condition which the negligence triggers, then the plaintiff is liable even though it is not foreseen by the defendant. For example, in *Smith v. Leech Brain & Co.* [1962] 2 QB 405, the plaintiff suffered a minor burn to his lip because of the defendant's negligence which activated an existing precancerous condition and he died. The defendant was liable – the employer only had to foresee that the plaintiff could suffer a burn, not that it could trigger a malignant condition.

Avoiding liability in negligence

Defences
There are situations in which, although the defendant has been negligent, s/he may avoid liability:

- *Limitation periods.* If a patient has suffered personal injury and wishes to bring a negligence action against the nurse or NHS Trust, then s/he must commence a legal action within three years from the time the damage occurred, or from when the defendant had knowledge of the cause of action. This three-year limit may be extended in the case of children until they are 21 years of age, and for mentally-disordered persons whilst their mental disorder prevents them from commencing the action. The time limit for other forms of damage is six years.
- *Contributory negligence.* This is not a complete defence, but may reduce the amount of damages which are payable when a nurse has been negligent (*Sayers* v. *Harlow Urban District Council* [1958] 1 WLR 623). Contributory negligence is relevant when the defendant is partly to blame for his own injuries, for example when a passenger in a car suffers injuries in a car crash and s/he has not worn a seat belt. The partial defence is rarely successful in medical negligence cases but could be relevant in family-centred care, for example if the parent deliberately and without the knowledge of the nursing staff departed from the agreed treatment plan. However, the nurse would still be liable if s/he was in breach of duty by inadequately

supervising the parent or s/he could be liable in negligence by wrongly delegating the child's treatment to a clearly unsuitable parent.

● *If one of the three elements of negligence cannot be proved,* for example if there is a break in the chain of causation. For example, if something unforeseen should happen, and as a result the child patient suffers injury, a new cause of the harm may be established which will prevent a finding of negligence against the nurse.

Documentation
Negligence actions may take years before they come to court and complex cases may take over ten years before they are concluded. Given this time scale it is highly likely that memories of events and conversations may become vague and distorted, and so it is essential that reliable records and documentation of treatment decisions and agreements between the nursing staff and parents concerning the care of the child are maintained. Records could be vital in establishing exactly what happened, and may determine whether negligence is proven. If there is uncertainty this could be to the plaintiff's advantage, since s/he must prove negligence on the balance of probabilities (more likely than not) and lack of firm evidence to the contrary may make negligence easier to establish. The documentation should include:

(i)   Whether the parents agree to take part in the care-by-parent scheme in the nursing care plan.
(ii)   What procedures the parents have agreed to undertake.
(iii)   What teaching has been undertaken.
(iv)   Whether parents are confident about taking on certain tasks in the hospital and at home.
(v)   A review of planned care with progress update.

Any additions or amendments to the care plan should be recorded, checked, signed and dated.

The parents' signature on the documentation does not legally establish that the parents have assumed the nurse's responsibility. The signature is only confirmation that the parents agree to participate in the care, have agreed to undertake a certain procedure, that they have been taught how to carry out that procedure, or that they feel confident in taking on specific tasks. It does not exempt the staff or the hospital from liability if they have been negligent in some way. Nor does it clarify sufficiently what the parent has been told or taught. In the event of a dispute it will still usually be a question of one person's word against another's. The requirement of a parent's signature may actually act against the aims of family-centred care as the parent may feel that responsibility is being shifted to him/her and that s/he is being abandoned by the professional staff. So rather than acting as a team with the uniform aim of the child's best interests, the requirement of a signature may act as a barrier, with parents on one side and the hospital staff on another.

Professional discipline

The nurse is not only accountable to his/her employer and to his/her patients by way of the law, but she is also accountable to the UKCC. The UKCC *Guidelines for Professional Practice* (1996) advise nurses that

> If you delegate work to someone who is not registered with the UKCC, your accountability is to make sure that the person who does the work is able to do it and that appropriate levels of supervision or support are in place.

Of course in addition to a nurse being held to be negligent s/he may also be at risk of having his/her right to practice taken away by the nurses' professional body, the UKCC. The Professional Conduct Committee is open to find a nurse guilty of misconduct and so remove him/her from the register. The professional conduct rules defines professional misconduct as 'conduct unworthy of a nurse, midwife or health visitor,' and in the past professional misconduct has included breach of confidentiality, a failure to keep records or falsifying records, and reckless and willfully unskilled practice. It is also possible that proceedings would be brought where a nurse fails to adhere to guidelines established by the employer. A nurse who has been negligent may be found guilty of misconduct and be removed from the register. A finding of professional misconduct differs from a finding of negligence in law, since it does not require proof of injury which is an essential requirement of negligence – proof of negligence or other misconduct is sufficient.

Gross negligence: criminal liability

If the conduct of the health professional amounts to gross negligence and a patient dies, then the practitioner could be prosecuted for gross negligence manslaughter (*R* v. *Adomako* [1995] 1 AC 171). Whether or not the defendant is considered sufficiently negligent that criminal liability should attach is a matter for the jury, but the current test is that a defendant is liable when s/he has shown such disregard for the life and safety of others as to deserve punishment (*R* v. *Batemen* (1925) 19 Cr App R 8). For a practitioner to be found grossly negligent, the three elements of negligence must be proved and also whether, 'having regard to the risk of death involved, [was] the conduct of the defendant ... so bad in all the circumstances as to amount to a criminal act or omission?' (*R* v. *Adomako* [1995] 1 AC 171, 187).

Occupiers' liability

The nurse may vicariously create liability for his/her employer on the basis of the NHS Trust's duty of care to visitors on its premises under the Occupiers' Liability Act 1957. This statute establishes that the occupier of premises owes a duty of care to its lawful visitors, which would include patients, their families, visitors and other employees. To comply with the duty of care, the Trust (as occupier) and its employees (as agents of the Trust) must ensure that they take

> such care as in all the circumstances of the case is reasonable to see that the visitor will be reasonably safe in using the premises for the purposes for which he is invited or permitted by the occupier to be there. (Section 2(2) Occupiers' Liability Act 1957)

Therefore the nurse must be constantly vigilant as to situations which may represent potential hazards to the child patient and their families who may be present on the ward 24 hours a day. The nurse should also be prepared for children to be less careful than adults, and so they must be accorded a higher degree of care (Section 2(3)(a) Occupiers' Liability Act 1957).

Summary

It is important that healthcare practitioners should be aware of their potential legal liability within their daily work. The current emphasis on patient autonomy, the concept of the patient as client, and the growth of the litigation culture should encourage practitioners to understand and be aware of the legal and professional implications of their actions. Family-centred care requires the same vigilance as other specialisms, but particular attention should be paid to the working relationship between practitioners and parents. Attention paid to communication with the parents and an understanding of their concerns and problems may resolve and prevent any misunderstandings or difficulties which could arise. Practitioners should also ensure that efficient and thorough documentation of the patient's care is maintained so as to resolve any potential factual uncertainties.

References

Dimond, B. (1990) 'Parental Acts and Omissions', *Paediatric Nursing*, February, 2(1), pp. 23–4.
Smith, F. (1995) *Children's Nursing in Practice: The Nottingham Model* (Oxford: Blackwell Science).
UKCC (1992) *Code of Professional Conduct, for the Nurse, Midwife and Health Visitor* (London: UKCC).
UKCC (1996) *Guidelines for Professional Practice* (London: UKCC).
UKCC (2000) *Guidelines for the Administration of Medicines* (London: UKCC).

Index